Caregiving, Carebots, and Contagion

REVOLUTIONARY BIOETHICS

Series Editor: Rachel Haliburton, University of Sudbury

Revolutionary Bioethics is a new series composed of scholarly monographs and edited collections organized around specific topics that explore bioethical theory and practice through the frameworks provided by feminist ethics, narrative ethics, and virtue ethics, challenging the assumptions of mainstream bioethics in the process. Contemporary mainstream bioethics has become ideological and repetitive, a defender of activities that bioethics was originally created to critique, and an apologist for unethical practices and policies in medicine that it once saw itself as fighting against. Taking its title from recent work being done on MacIntyre's neo-Aristotelian ethics, Revolutionary Bioethics is organized around the idea that bioethics needs to reform both its theory and practice, and its goal is to begin the conversation about what a transformed bioethics—one that is unafraid to explore new theoretical approaches, and to examine and critique current bioethical practices—might look like.

Titles in the series

Caregiving, Carebots, and Contagion, by Michael C. Brannigan

Engineering Perfection: Solidarity, Disability, and Well-being, by Elyse Purcell

Physician-Assisted Suicide and Euthanasia: Before, During, and After the Third Reich, edited by Sheldon Rubenfeld and Daniel P. Sulmasy, with Astrid Ley

Caregiving, Carebots, and Contagion

Michael C. Brannigan

LEXINGTON BOOKS
Lanham • Boulder • New York • London

Published by Lexington Books
An imprint of The Rowman & Littlefield Publishing Group, Inc.
4501 Forbes Boulevard, Suite 200, Lanham, Maryland 20706
www.rowman.com

86-90 Paul Street, London EC2A 4NE

Copyright © 2022 by The Rowman & Littlefield Publishing Group, Inc.

All rights reserved. No part of this book may be reproduced in any form or by any electronic or mechanical means, including information storage and retrieval systems, without written permission from the publisher, except by a reviewer who may quote passages in a review.

British Library Cataloguing in Publication Information Available

Library of Congress Cataloging-in-Publication Data On File

ISBN 978-1-7936-4918-8 (cloth)
ISBN 978-1-7936-4920-1 (pbk.)
ISBN 978-1-7936-4919-5 (electronic)

*To my dear friend Kay Toombs, philosopher extraordinaire,
who personally knows full well the power of caregiving.
Her love and kindness is a deep river.*

Contents

Acknowledgments	ix
Introduction: Then, Now, and To Come	xiii
Chapter One: Are Robots Made for This?	1
Chapter Two: Promise	21
Chapter Three: Peril	45
Chapter Four: What Is in a Face?	73
Chapter Five: Poise	97
Bibliography	121
Index	133
About the Author	145

Acknowledgments

One stubborn irony behind this book is that while its ultimate theme pares down to an urgent call for physical, face-to-face engagement, I have composed it during these times necessitating the opposite. Its message of resuscitating presence, however, was sparked well before our purgatory of absence. Providentially for me, the absence was corporal, not personal. Family, friends, and colleagues have not remained socially distant—the official, though at times wrongheaded rubric. They have shown their unfaltering support despite our separate dispersions. To them all, I remain forever grateful for cheering me on and for the edifying lessons they have shown in what it means to care. They are all close to heart and mind.

First, our beloved parents, mine and Brooke's—Misae, Tom, Del, and Carl—have each departed over a brief stretch of four years. They never stopped loving us, wishing we always live good lives, and being our first teachers of the nature of caring. My dear sisters Maggie and Marie, twins and dancing artists, are ever-devoted to family, friends, students, and their graceful calling. As for vocations, my treasured brother Tom was clearly born to be a caregiver, which he lives out in noble, selfless fashion. Brooke gave her all in caring for her brother Ken, who departed a few years after our parents. Ken too lived selflessly in giving to his children Dan and Kate.

Miracles and magic await our newly married nephew Dan and niece Kate as they journey forth from their new beginnings: Dan with Stephanie and their newborn, pretty Sarah Rose, and Kate with Kyle. May their new shores be filled with godsends. When it comes to family, we cannot forget Julia Schilling, our treasured German "daughter" who, with all her kin, ever since we met in tiny Altenschwand, always occupy a special, huge room in our home and hearts. Skip and Mary Rosa, without any doubt one of the best fortunes to bless the Brannigan clan—always give, always care. The same goes for my cousin David and his cherished new bride Jess. May theirs be a celestial match that will paddle through whatever currents the seas impart.

The same goes for newlyweds Tad Connerton and Stephanie Schwetz, Jim Fanning and Deana Miller. My lifelong buddies Tad and Jim are now in better hands, and their lives so much richer. Tad and Stephanie sharing with us via Zoom chats, good wine, and music. Jim and Deana with their abiding faith and humor. All have sturdily showered Brooke and me with their love and grace. Ever since we met at the University of Leuven and played music together in our little band, Cliff Muldoon has shared in the challenging journey inward in the spirit of the Middle Way. Cliff's support is solid, exuding honor and character.

Dr. Mark and Kathy Sullivan are always there in our corner, through all seasons, unsullied. They and their clan extraordinaire are purer than Irish mist. Their bond remains unfailing. Marilyn Presto, my precious friend and bona fide former leader at the helm of the University of Missouri-Kansas City's sterling Bioethics and Humanities program, embodies presence with her smile, quiet, and calm. Dr. Frank McCluskey, Zen sensei and my lifelong partner in our philosophical dig, along with his wonderful bride Melanie, remain unflappable friends. And there is Dr. Kim Grego and Jack, and Dr. Alessandra Vincentini with her Andrea and Giuliano. Kim and Alessandra have always shown their unswerving support as they move forward in their marvelous pioneering work in recognizing the plight of caregiving and elders worldwide. My dear friend Dr. Antoinette Fage-Butler, whose Irish grace and wisdom has always blessed me, as she in turn is blessed by her beautiful family in Denmark, is never without a kind word.

Our treasured companions Paul and Eileen Churchill unaffectedly incarnate a deep wellspring of kindness, wisdom, and bigheartedness without limit, as friendship should be. They are gifts to all who know them. Doctors Bonnie Gray and Ari Greyson, whose friendship is unbroken, untainted, are always there with kind hearts, comfort, reassurance, and keen grasp of Japanese insight and good sake. And Diana Grillo and Erik Carlson remain faithful friends who never fail in offering us their warm greetings and support. They are a perfect blend of Italian zest and Viking grit. Setsuko Matsuyama, my Japanese colleague and "sister," along with cherished Hiroko, Kunio, and Izumi live always in my soul as does my homeland. As do numerous others, Japanese and Irish cousins and friends, voices with their epistles, faces with their epiphanies. Our webs of *aidagara*, "in-between," run deep. Though unnamed, they too live in my heart. A special cheer to Molly Sager and her precious family. Even through gauntlets they've weathered, they remain hopeful, giving, and committed to élan vital. My goddaughter Kelly is ever a guiding star for her family and lads Conor and Graham, never failing to inspire. I offer my appreciation to Dr. Craig Condella, chair of Salve Regina University's Philosophy department, whom I've not yet met personally, but has steadily encouraged me since I've joined their team. So also Jay

Jochnowitz, good friend and esteemed editor at the *Albany Times Union*, also a humble connoisseur of the demanding art of *kyudo*, has been always generous in granting me reprieve to work on this book.

This is not my first book with editor-in-chief Jana Hodges-Kluck. Indeed, I remain blessed and genuinely grateful for her expertise, professionalism, direction, and positivity. Jana is the model editor. She calls it like it is, without fluff. At the same time, she graciously reassures every step of the way. And to get this project off the ground, that's a lot of steps. You know a leader by the staff she appoints. Sydney Wedbush never fails in responding to my questions super-promptly and with encouragement and know-how. And Professor Rachel Haliburton has placed her confidence in my project for her innovative and much-needed Revolutionary Bioethics series. Neither is this my first work with Diane Brenner as trusty indexer. Whenever I check out a new book, I first check out the index. Diane, with her keen eye for thematic matter and expertise, comes through with sterling work. To her, I am always grateful. My gratitude also to my reviewer who has offered most helpful comments and insights. We need thoughtful perspectives of others who can save us from ourselves.

Time in research and writing takes away time from family and friends. During this protracted COVID limbo, time assumes an added existential cadence as we struggle to use it to stay connected with those dear to us. Hopefully, we have also awakened to what really counts. Along these lines, this brings me to my beautiful wife, life-companion and lighthouse Brooke. She has, over the years, stayed steady, ever-patient, tolerant of my moods, keeping serene through the delights we have discovered and storms we have weathered, reminding me of what matters. I will never live enough lifetimes to show her my love.

Introduction

Then, Now, and To Come

THEN

The scourge came swiftly. Life Care Center of Kirkland, Washington, had its first COVID-19 casualty in late February 2020. After just four weeks, its death toll from the contagion climbed to over 30. For nursing homes, a sign of things to come. The numbers stayed grim. In the first four months of the pathogen's entry into the U.S., over 50,000 long-term care residents and workers died from the novel coronavirus. Settings included assisted living and skilled nursing quarters. The fatality rate stayed steady through December 2020, totaling nearly 100,000 deaths, over 43 percent of all deaths in the country. Yet less than 1 percent of the U.S. population are nursing home residents.[1] Likewise, global long-term care fatalities from the disease were strikingly lopsided compared to countries' overall death toll. As of August 11, 2020, U.S. nursing home deaths represented 42 percent of the country's total number; in Belgium they constituted 49 percent; 46 percent in France; 54 percent in Ireland; 66 percent in Australia; 78 percent in Canada; 39 percent in Germany; 37 percent in Italy; and 68 percent in Spain.[2] All this strikes at the disproportionality of victims in nursing homes.

The wounds were unspeakably heart-wrenching as residents and workers died alone, their loved ones helplessly waiting and wondering. Allison Lolley's 81-year-old mother Cheryl, a resident in a nursing home in Monroe, Louisiana, was a victim. Prohibited from visiting her mother, Allison would often see her through the window. "Our family watched Mama deteriorate. She complained of lack of care, and 'manhandling' from people in her room that she didn't recognize. During one visit to her window, I found Mama unclothed, unkempt, and confused. I reported these issues and received boilerplate explanations or promises to handle it "immediately."[3] Nursing home staff too watched and waited, with little in the way of personal protective equipment (PPE), medical resources, and guidance from federal, state, and local officials. Sherry Perry, a certified nursing assistant at a long-term care site in Lebanon, Tennessee put it bluntly. "They locked the doors, and it was on us to figure things out. Thirty years on the job and I was now flying blind. These residents touch us. We roll them, toilet them, take care of them. You can't really social distance in a nursing home."[4]

The Real Epicenter

Nursing homes were the real epicenter of the pandemic. Why? Not only are nursing homes the *de facto* option for elders. Consider residents' medical status. Many are functionally disabled, powerless to engage in regular daily activities. Many suffer from debilitating forms of cognitive impairment. Nearly all residents endure chronic comorbidities like hypertension as well as cardiovascular, respiratory, and neurological diseases, dementia, stroke, diabetes, and various malignancies. These conditions require sustained physical interaction between workers and residents, with increased exposure to infection. Moreover, now and in the future, residents will suffer long-term outcomes of the pandemic, harsh declines in mental health, and swelling tides of hopelessness.[5]

Nursing homes do not exist in bubbles. Every long-term care facility networks with other settings, and those in turn connect with clusters of others like homeless shelters, contracting companies, and food processing plants. This sets the stage for steady outbreaks. In addition to patient transfers, vital workers like facility crews, physicians, nurses, drivers, dialysis technicians, hospice staff, and chaplains regularly come in and out of nursing homes. And with mounting understaffing, multiple agencies offer on-call nursing services for these and the expanding chains of nursing home affiliates. Here we see the dark side of interconnection. For example, in one Florida nursing home "Not only is this facility directly linked to 52 other homes—substantially higher than the state's average of 11.4—many of these direct connections are themselves highly connected, demonstrating the importance of capturing the entire network in these outcome measures."[6] These links played a major role in nursing home outbreaks. Visits to multiple long-term care settings in many cases likely transmitted the virus. This was worsened with patient transfers to other facilities. Given the over 15,000 nursing homes in the U.S., worker mobility and patient transfers undoubtedly played a major role in nursing home outbreaks. One insightful analysis used device-level location data over an 11-week period from over 500,000 smartphones of nursing home staff and contractors. It found that over 5 percent of users visited other long-term care facilities. The report concludes:

Introduction xv

> While our methodology cannot establish causation, we find that the number and strength of connections between nursing homes—and a home's centrality within the greater network—strongly predict Covid cases, even after controlling for location, demographic factors, number of beds, for-profit status, and CMS [Centers for Medicare & Medicaid Services] quality ratings.[7]

With nursing staff employed at multiple nursing homes, contagion more easily spread. "With an estimated 49% of nursing home cases attributable to cross-facility staff movement, attention to highly connected nursing homes is warranted."[8]

Scandalous understaffing was a glaring issue well before the pandemic. This, along with so many clusters of affiliations and networks, inevitably generated shared staffing. To support their families, many staff would work in different nursing homes, moving from one to the other. When COVID-19 hit, without a coordinated response, the workers were ill-prepared for the lethality and scope of the contagion. Furthermore, insufficient staffing combined with shoddy training for nurse aides. Attorney with the Center for Medicare Advocacy Toby Edelman cites this issue of substandard training.

> The situation in nursing homes became horrible. Overnight we lost transparency and accountability. After CMS waived the 75-hour training requirement for nurse aides, many states allowed staff to provide care after just an eight-hour online training program. Workers are sick, they're dying, taking care of their own families. New staff are needed because residents need care. But eight hours?[9]

Predictably, the blame game ran full speed from the start. Amid the finger-pointing and deplorable lack of accountability, prominent facts stand out. There was virtually no understanding of the likelihood of asymptomatic transmission. Federal and state relief was meager. Information regarding the scope of impact on elders was sparse. Caregivers encountered an appallingly dire lack of personal protective equipment. There were no efforts toward long-term care institutional testing. When the Centers for Medicare & Medicaid Services eventually required testing in nursing homes in September, it was far too late. Things became even worse when lockdown measures barred nursing home inspectors as well as residents' ombudsmen. Communication between nursing homes and residents' families was dismal. Symptomatic residents' were at times refused admission to hospital emergency rooms.[10] Frankly, nursing homes were blatantly not a priority.[11] This deprioritizing of long-term care facilities unambiguously reflects how ageism in America is alive and well. AARP's (American Association of Retired Persons) VP of government affairs for state advocacy Elaine Ryan highlights how this was apparent after initial lockdowns. "It was stunning to see that at the start of the pandemic, there was quick action to dismiss college students from campuses, to close down basketball games because these were congregate settings. Yet nursing home residents were ignored. No one suggested moving them to safer settings. As I see it, the problem was ageism."[12]

NOW

With the staggering number of COVID-19 related deaths in nursing facilities worldwide, residents dying alone, caregivers worn to the bone facing the ongoing threat of infection, we can turn to our machines for help and relief. Enter the robots. Surely, health professionals and caregivers will be the ones working closest to and with their patients and residents, *for now*. However, caring robots will step in with a wide range of functional assistance. Whether we can alter our consumerist dispositions and ecological plundering remains in doubt. What is certain is that robotic technologies will assume a major, perhaps dominant, role in our nursing and healthcare facilities. Caring robots, or what philosopher Shannon Vallor calls "carebots," are being designed to assist, support, and offer care for elders, sick, disabled, young, and other vulnerable groups.[13] It is almost as if they were made for this. According to a *Boston Globe* headline in 2014, robots are this century's "newest must-study subject," and books, articles, and blogs are pounded out at super speed. The newest prototypes have a short life, swiftly outdated with newer models. Research rushes on, unstoppable, as in the film "Matrix" scene when Agent Smith wrestles with Neo on the railway tracks. As a fast-moving train approaches, Smith says, "You hear that Mr. Anderson? That is the sound of inevitability." Robots are the inevitable result of the nonstop and persistent development, design, and progress in artificial intelligence (AI) and robotics.

Like the train, advances in AI in medicine proceed full steam, progressing considerably in its applications having learned decisive lessons since IBM's supercomputer Watson Health. Watson's learning capacity to cull through millions of pages of medical literature and research, mining medical data from patients' images and family histories, and forming and testing hypotheses from the data promised sound treatment recommendations. It overreached in its ambitious effort to come up with cures for the complex constellation of cancer. Yet upon forming partnerships with healthcare titans like Mayo Clinic, Sloan Kettering, and Johnson & Johnson, it achieved prominent triumphs as well as defeats. One triumph was its work with the University of North Carolina's Lineberger Comprehensive Cancer Center when Watson recommended appropriate clinical trials for over 300 patients, trials that were initially missed by their oncologists.[14] IBM's work with MD Anderson, however, was not successful. Cardiologist Eric Topol describes the venture as "a debacle noteworthy for many missteps. One of the most fundamental was the claim that ingesting millions of pages of medical information was the same as being able to make sense, or use, of the information."[15] We continue to insist that humans still do the processing and sense-making when it comes to specifics like interpreting electrocardiograms (EKGs), pathology slides, imaging tests and scans. But the machine is definitely gaining ground. For instance, in the quirky terrain of predictability, a collaborative venture between Mayo Clinic and the AI company AliveCor are working on how close a smartwatch can come to detect high potassium (K+) blood levels that could lead to disorders such as heart arrhythmias.[15]

The marriage of AI and robotics has unambiguously paved the way for robots. Note AI expert Takanori Shibata's baby harp seal Paro. "Paro" is shorthand for *pāsonaru robotto*, the Japanese pronunciation of "personal robot." Paro performs effectively as a "mental assistant robot" and a therapeutic pet companion for elders in nursing homes, hospitals, and in their own home settings. Paro moves its eyes, eyelids, and its head, emits cries in response to human touch and voice. It knows its name. It reacts to noises and senses the softness and roughness of a touch. Because of its lifelike response to persons being cared-for, Paro's effect on their physical and mental well-being has been positive. It has enhanced users' cognitive skills, reduced their stress and depression, and has helped to smooth the way for more positive interaction between users and other humans. It surely provides comfort for hospitalized children. Its mere presence is supportive. Although Paro does not actively facilitate human-to-human interaction, by simply being-there, it is a conduit for this to come about.

A carebot is there, ready-at-hand, present to the cared-for and this means a lot. It is reassuring to know the carebot is there, but not obtrusive. Kazuo Ishiguro's recent novel *Klara and the Sun* is a delightfully thoughtful romp into a future when sociable robots, "artificial friends," or "AF," are *au courant*.[17] Written from the first-person perspective of Klara, the tale centers on the unfolding friendship between a sick girl, Josie, and her solar-powered AF, Klara. It also describes the relationship between Klara and Josie's boyfriend, Rick, and her mother. As soon as she spots Klara on display at a store selling artificial friends, Josie feels immediately drawn to it. Though newer AF prototypes are more popular, Klara shows exceptional perception, sensitivity, and hints of empathy. When Josie stops by the storefront window with her mother and sees Klara the second time, she asks Klara if Klara would like to come home with her. Klara nods supportively. Josie is thrilled, but wants to share with Klara that it may be challenging at times because of her illness.

> "Listen," she said . . . "It's so great you want to come. But I want things straight between us from the start, so I'm going to say this. Don't worry, Mom can't

hear. Look, I think you'll like our house. I think you'll like my room, and that's where you'll be, not in some cupboard or anything. And we'll do all those great things together all the time I'm growing up. Only thing is, sometimes, well . . . " She glanced back quickly again, then lowering her voice further, said: "Maybe it's because some days I'm not so well. I don't know. But there might be something going on. I'm not sure what it is. I don't even know if it's something bad. But things sometimes get, well, unusual. Don't get me wrong, most times you wouldn't feel it. But I wanted to be straight with you. Because you know how lousy it feels, people telling you how perfect things will be and they're not being straight. Please say you still want to come . . . "

I nodded to her through the glass, as seriously as I knew how. I also wanted to tell her that if there was anything difficult, anything frightening, to be faced in her house, we could do so together. But I didn't know how to convey such a complex message through the glass without words, and so I clasped my hands together and held them up, shaking them slightly, in a gesture I'd seen a taxi driver give from inside his moving taxi to someone who'd waved from the sidewalk, even though he had to take both hands off his steering wheel. Whatever Josie understood from it, it seemed to make her happy.[18]

Throughout the story, Klara senses when to be conspicuous and when to be discreet. But is this being-present, ready-at-hand, the same as human presence? Is the carebot's presence its own? Can human presence be replicated, the presence that comes with active listening, genuine seeing, gut feeling, intuition, empathy, compassion, and especially that precious human feature—the capacity to imagine? Imagination is the runway to empathy. Only by imagining another's plight can we inch closer to feeling it. Philosopher Kay Toombs evocatively underscores this link between imagination and empathy.

> It is clear that if one is to attempt to grasp experiences so unlike one's own, one must have the capacity to *imagine* what it might be like. And, indeed, *imagination* is integral to the task of understanding the meaning of illness-as-lived. If one is to come to some understanding of the patient's meanings, interpretations, values, and so forth, it is essential to grasp (as nearly as possible) what it is like for the other person to be in this particular situation.[19]

Human-robot interaction surely affects human-human interaction, and vice versa. The more we desocialize our human interaction, the more we open the door to allow the machine to substitute for the human. Humans, certainly less reliable, are less needed.

The worst enemy is one who has nothing to lose, has no fear of dying. And when the enemy is unseen and everywhere, no armed might can defeat it. Our only weapon lies in our reason, wits, and will. Those on the frontlines in hospitals, long-term care settings, manufacturing, pharmacies, police, fire and rescue units, etc. who do their jobs and whatever it takes to keep us safe have shown us those traits of reason, wits, and will. On the other hand, we have witnessed more than enough signs of doltish, reckless, opportunistic, and self-centered responses to this global contagion. These are our internal threats. How will we face our external threats such as the dangerous changes in climate spurring on recurrent extreme weather, and further outbreaks of infectious diseases? In the ever-shifting gale winds of pathological microbes and dangerously mutating viruses, the one constancy is the threat of contagion. To deal with this threat, in the intrinsically human vocation of medicine, robots can wonderfully aid and assist patients and caregivers.

While carebots offer lifesaving promises for our future, perils accompany their promises. We will explore both promises and perils. Technological interventions, particularly in healthcare communication, have become the rule of thumb, replacing interpersonal, embodied, face-to-face interaction. They have a hold over us, offering us the lure of the new, the quick fix, efficiency, sense of control, and feelings of certainty. In particular, carebots confer a sense of safety and security, so desperately needed in our increasingly precarious and lonely world. Yet, while carebots may offer a sheltered zone protecting us from the uncertainties and infection that come with human-to-human encounters, problems arise should they replace human caring. When we view our machines as "fixes," we further estrange ourselves from embodied, person-to-person, face-to-face interaction. This will produce unintended side effects that diminish our own capacities as humans.

The benefits of caring robots are enormous and life-saving. At the same time, they raise profound moral and existential questions. Can carebots *replace* human caring? Can they offer empathy and compassion? What does it mean to care? What kind of society will we shape? What does it mean to be human? This book is not about the newest technologies and state-of-the-art prototypes. Philosophical and existentially moral in design, it seeks to address deep-rooted, intimate questions as to who we are as humans, how we relate to others, and what society we wish to inhabit in the near and distant future. My claim in the following pages is straightforward. While carebots can provide undeniable hands-on benefits in caring for elders, disabled, and other vulnerable groups, particularly during times of contagion, caring, at its core, is a fundamentally human act. Caring lies at the heart of ethics. As humans, we have a fundamental moral responsibility to care for the Other. And genuine caring demands an embodied, person-to-person, flesh and bone presence with the Other.

TO COME

Scientists have warned us of pandemics to come. Epidemiologists and other infectious disease experts have steadily sounded the alarm. Noted virologist Michael B. A. Oldstone cautioned us over two decades ago: "Of the plagues that visit humans, influenza is among those that require constant surveillance, because we can be certain that some form of influenza will continue to return."[20] We share in the precarious chemistry of ecology, climate threats, human incursions into the natural world, and resulting zoonotic diseases whereby "a pathogen leaps from some nonhuman animal into a person, and succeeds there in establishing itself as an infectious presence," notes science writer David Quammen.[21] And because of our continued human-wildlife interfacing, veterinary infectious disease expert Eric Fèvre warns us that "New diseases pop-up in the human population probably three to four times per year . . . It's not just in Asia or Africa, but in Europe and the US as well . . . This kind of event is likely to happen again and again."[22] And we have stubbornly plugged our ears, sadly unprepared in past outbreaks. How prepared are we now and into the future? What about our drug manufacturing infrastructure? Is it ready to deal with national crises and shortages? A study at University of Minnesota's Center for Infectious Disease Research and Policy (CIDRAP) surveyed pharmacists pertaining to the most critical must-need drugs, "drugs they absolutely had to have on a day-to-day basis. Not cancer drugs, not AIDS drugs, but the essential, needed-to-sustain-life-can't-wait-until-tomorrow drug." The center's director Michael T. Osterholm and author/filmmaker Mark Olshaker compiled their listing. This study, conducted just prior to the 2009 H1N1, swine flu, outbreak, consisted of over 30 crucial pharmacological agents, including:

> Insulin for type 1 diabetics; the vasodilator nitroglycerine; heparin for blood thinning and dialysis; succinylcholine for muscle relaxation during surgery, intubation, and heart-lung machine hookup; Lasix for congestive heart failure; metaprolol for angina and severe hypertension; norepinephrine for severe hypotension; albuterol to open airways in the lungs; and various other heart and blood circulatory drugs and basic antibiotics.[23]

How many of these drugs were manufactured in the U.S.? Their finding: "One hundred percent of these drugs were generic; all were manufactured primarily or exclusively overseas, mostly in India and China; there were no significant stockpiles, and the supply chains were long and extremely vulnerable."[24] As for the future, they assert that "influenza is hyperevolving, more so than at any other time in the earth's history. The huge number of animals needed to produce our food serves as the amplifying factor for virus transmission and, in turn, for more spins at the genetic roulette table."[25]

Can We Stretch Our Time-Scope?

Along with this need to be suitably prepared, there is another, more human, challenge. We humans face an inordinate hurdle in our precarious inability to stretch our temporal horizon, our time-scope, enough to conceptualize and imagine ourselves in a distant, though near enough, future. We are not solely beings-toward-our-own deaths. Martin Heidegger's vista is certainly on target to a degree. However, as Emmanuel Levinas reminds us, we exist toward a time *beyond* our departure. That is our perennial task—to see further than our personal, temporal skyline. Can we place ourselves in a future 50, 100 years from now? We can surely imagine what it might be like, a time nearly given over to super-enhanced AI and robotics, a time in which the human-machine interface is so indelibly interwoven that it is difficult to distinguish the two. This kind of conceptualizing lies in my imaginings, a future for others and future others. However, I still do not belong to it. I remain a detached observer of a future 'not mine' so that this diminishes my engagement with the idea, the thoughts, the imaginings. It is less real for me than my five years from now in which I can more tangibly visualize my living, playing tennis, sea kayaking, writing, being with Brooke, awakening together and embracing each day's promises. In the same way, we humans lack the capacity to think of long-term in the same way we visualize the soon-to-come. Our futures are dim, high-level cirrus clouds, above 20,000 feet. Thus, the invaluable teacher we call history. To better glimpse our future, know the past. And when it comes to future storms, how we deal with them rests on how we are *before* the storm.

Not long ago, mechanical elevators gradually replaced nearly all human elevator operators, a virtually extinct occupation except in those few hotels holding on to the tradition of making the ride up and down less isolated, at least prior to Covid. In our human-machine interface, we have traveled the expected slim Hegelian cycle of response—first reacting with trepidation, fear, and concern, to gradual acceptance through practice and subsequent habit. Now that we have gone from bulky industrial robots to mobile military bots for bomb disposal, surveillance, being weapons, and more recently to "social" robots as guides in shopping malls, hospitals, and as companions in nursing homes, we have further reason to ask: What does the future bode regarding our human-machine interaction? While we can leave that question to the futurists among us as well as to those technicians, engineers, and scientists in the trenches here and now, my concern is existential and moral, dosed with reasoned speculation. With our heightening human-robot interaction, what are the implications regarding caring for human beings? Is caring for another human at its root and essence a distinctively human affair, and therefore a fallible act and state of mind?

In System We Trust

There is much to be said of fallibility. Fallibility captures the bottom line of our humanness. We are built to create, invent, and produce. We are also built to make mistakes. We humans make amazing, life-changing, life-saving discoveries. We paint our starry nights and compose music that reaches the heavens, like Rachmaninoff's Symphony 2, third movement's Adagio. But we also make horrific mistakes and bad decisions, abuse and murder living beings. We generate, willfully or not, misery. Worldwide, we kill over 1.2 million of each other on the road with our vehicles every year. With all our hype over driverless cars, we get bent out of shape when an autonomous car kills a human. We have conditioned ourselves to blindly trust the system that produced the car. After investigation, it was determined that the first fatality from a driverless car was the result of human error. In the 2018 Uber robot car crash in Tempe, Arizona, the human "safety driver" paid more attention to her phone.[26] Though we cannot count on our digital systems to monitor for ethical lapses, we still trust the systems behind Google, Amazon, Facebook, Apple, Microsoft and other super-tech giants to do their thing. We selectively choose which fallibility to remedy: machines rather than humans. As we will see, uncritical trust in the system behind digital health can spell disaster.

To be sure the time has not arrived, not yet. But that does not mean we ought to wait until that time comes and then deal with it. Expectation precedes preparation. We must be able to anticipate a scenario that may never unfold. In so doing, we need to reflect on what that means regarding how we think of ourselves as humans, how we relate to other humans, and how we relate to our machines. To glimpse the future, we open our eyes to the now. The late Warner Slack of Harvard Medical School asserted, "If a physician can be replaced by a computer, then he or she deserves to be replaced by a computer."[27] Rightly the same can be said concerning caregivers. If they can be replaced by robots, then they should. What does this say apropos the nature of caring? Will machines eventually replace specialists like the radiologist, dermatologist, ophthalmologist, oncologist, surgeon, or therapist? The response is mixed. Some feel robots will complement and enhance the specialist's work. With robot therapists and companions, will we prefer conditioned fantasies of emotion and empathy? It is cleaner, neither murky nor soiled from human complexities of the ilk that have us escape into our silos. Or will our human-robot interaction lead to richer, more enduring human-to-human interaction? As a robot companion baby seal sparks conversation among nursing home residents who were formerly entrenched in their solitariness, each waiting for a visitor. In truth, how we engage with our robots reveals much about ourselves, like our desire to want it all, the help without the hassles. We want our companions, servants, helpers, and slaves though without the rebellion in Karel Čapek's "R.U.R." and in Philip K. Dick's *Do Androids Dream of Electric Sheep?* We desire our robots to be autonomous only to a degree. Yet, should that time come when it is customary to consult with our robot therapist, or hire a hospice robot, or, even worse, tip our robot waiter or porter, we have sunk deeper into the rabbit hole. On the way down, we have shattered the irreducible hiddenness in both our solitariness and togetherness, the source of our laughter, tears, embarrassment, shame, and choice to either bear with the potholes or commit suicide. When robot physicians deliver to us our diagnoses and prognoses, we have descended even further. Delivering bad news is a skill no algorithm can capture. It is an unfinished act of self-extinguishing as the doctor gives part of oneself away each time he or she delivers the news. It eats one from the inside. The only glue that keeps the messenger in one piece is the human connection, a bridge built from lived-experience, a history that a caring robot would not have. Psychologist John Cohen was on to something nearly five decades ago when he wrote, "It would seem that at least three things characteristically human are out of reach of contemporary automata. In the first place, they are incapable of laughter (or tears); secondly, they do not blush; thirdly, they do not commit suicide."[28]

There will come a time when this global contagion is over. When we can breathe a collective sigh. But have no doubt, infectious pathogens are still alive. They never sleep. They seek new hosts. That is their nature. As events unfolded throughout our pandemic with lockdowns, riots, and politicizing of plain common sense, it has become all the more evident that, as a society, we have lost the critical capacity for nuance. We choose to see matters in white and black, either-or, red or blue. Where is our tolerance for complexity, for ambiguity, for uncertainty? Beyond any doubt, the human act of caregiving, while noble in its aim, is packed with complexities and uncertainties, particularly in circumstances of lethal contagion. Particularly when family members are the caregivers. Besides pathogenic perils, there are those muddy dynamics of human relationships. Human are not always reliable. In contrast, the hallmark of caring robots is their dependable performance. They act in ways that are caring. They see, hear, speak, clean, monitor, lift, wash, take vital signs, and respond to users' touch and voice. Will performance be good enough? That, in substance, is the core question that sparks all other questions I raise in this book. Here is an outline of my approach.

Outline

Each chapter starts with a brief retelling of an age-old and familiar Greek myth or legend. The reason is simple. Our visions of the boons of technologies we craft are imbedded in our veins. We desire to recreate ourselves and augment our powers in bold ways. Just as our imagination is a potential bridge to empathy, thereby a defining mark of what distinguishes us from robots, it also gives birth to universal parables of godly inspired artificial life. We not only dream of self-design and power, but make these dreams come alive, imprinting a natural kinship between myth, science, and technology. We are dreamers, doers, and makers who instinctively reach beyond our limits. But, as myths reveal, we pay a heavy price for the marvels we fashion. The legend of Prometheus has us formed from earth and water. But, as in Aesop's account, we come from earth and tears.

What has been compellingly evident throughout our pandemic is how intuitively Facetime, Skype, and Zoom became our default avenues to link up with each other. Chapter 1 makes it clear that our human-machine interface is nothing new, and robots have been around. Ongoing advances in artificial intelligence and robotics continue to extend our human capabilities. And in view of COVID-19's highly contagious nature, likely future pandemics, a rapidly aging world population, and the glaring deficit of caregivers, robots will no doubt be propelled into medicine's and caregiving's front lines. In many respects, they were made for this, as we shall see in full-throttle efforts to design robots to assist in caring in the U.S., Japan, and elsewhere. At the same time, we raise questions as to whether AI can solve the fundamental test, the "Riddle," of medical diagnosis. This summons us to ponder the possibility that super intelligent robots might someday replace medical specialists and human caregivers.

Robots offer numerous, far-reaching benefits when it comes to caregiving. Chapter 2 describes their invaluable promise, particularly during times of contagion. They can perform tasks that relieve caregivers' burden. On-call 24/7, requiring neither costly personal protective equipment nor health insurance, they can facilitate telemedicine, disinfect areas, take vital signs, deliver medicines, bring food, and help with boundary and distance control. In this way, they can save lives especially in high-stakes settings such as ships, prisons, and among the homeless. They can also assume more social and healing roles as companions and therapists.

We explore how AI has paved the way for caring robots and bot therapists. They are the inevitable result of our long history of human-machine interface. Steadily upgraded, carebots will no doubt complement, enlarge, and extend the benefits of human work with patients, particularly frail elderly, children and adults with autism spectrum disorder, and other vulnerable persons.

Grounded as these applications are in complex algorithms that seek to replicate human thinking and behavior, we then pose the question as to whether an algorithm can capture the involved dynamics of caregiving.

Technologies are often two-edged: they give and they take away. Despite their lifesaving promise, carebots present certain perils. Chapter 3 explores these. Technological interventions, particularly in healthcare communication, have become the rule of thumb, displacing interpersonal, embodied, face-to-face interaction. We explore this with a case study depicting adverse consequences from uncritical trust in digitized medicine. I describe the hold that new technologies have over us through the lure of the quick fix, efficiency, illusion of control, and feelings of certainty. While carebots offer a sense of safety and security, whether they can replace human caring, the nature of which we explore, is of crucial concern. *Taking care of* someone is not the same as *caring for* or *about* that person. *Taking care of*, what robots do, is caring as behavior, performance. It is radically distinct from caring as *caring for*, a feeling, attitude, and condition. Ultimately, in light of what genuine caring involves, should we consider our machines as fixes, we further estrange ourselves from embodied presence with each other. This, in turn, diminishes our humanness.

Carebots unequivocally illustrate our human-machine *interface*. What if they look human? If they have human faces? We address this in chapter 4. The deliberate design of robots as "companions" and "sociable robots," particularly in view of bold efforts to design 'self-conscious' robots, presents weighty challenges. Designing them to perform as companions involves the likely prospect of creating caring robots to appear and behave more like humans and with human faces. Will this make their caring more humanlike? More humane?

Here, we enter the dark terrain of the so-called uncanny valley, when a robot's human likeness crosses a line in which affect and interaction become eerie, non-human. The more human a robot seems, will its performance of caring be sufficient? My claim throughout this book is that it will not, for genuine caring and connectedness demands an embodied presence with others. All this not only makes us examine the true nature of caring, but raises questions regarding the meaning of the human face. Using insights from Maurice Merleau-Ponty, I describe the spirited uniqueness of human proximity and gesture. We then explore Emmanuel Levinas' remarkable vision of the meaning of the face, *le visage*, in that the encounter with a human face is extraordinarily singular and, in essence, a moral event. Along these lines, I argue that the human, flesh-and-blood face that both reveals and conceals remains indelibly unique and cannot be simulated.

Given our overreliance on machines, can we genuinely communicate with each other in ways that cultivate caring, or connectedness? Any sound resolution is not an either-or. Instead, we desperately need to strike a reasonable balance, to regain poise in our human-device interaction. In our final chapter, we address how we can sensibly pursue such poise and symmetry not only in how we interact with robots but more generally in our human-to-machine and human-to-human engagement. How we interface with our devices sets the tone for how we relate to ourselves and with each other. Carebots are not the culprits. Instead, the problem lies in *how we relate to them*. We need to learn to work together with them, to use them in ways that most beneficially complement our caregiving, in ways that empower us to further our own skill and art of genuine caring. I propose that caring is, *at its core*, our most noble human vocation. Of course it requires safe and skilled caregiving acts, acts that carebots can perform. At its heart, however, caring requires courage, empathy, communication, and embodied presence. I lay out ways to poise through moral machine design, embracing human singularity and aging, and cultivating embodied presence through listening, empathy, and our most human sense—touch. We conclude with a challenge of utmost urgency. We humans must achieve poise with our machines so that they supplement, not replace, our caregiving in ways that free us up to become better caregivers and enhance our ability to be more present with each other.

Our quest to recreate ourselves in our image is another version of Robert Jay Lifton's classic symbolic modes of immortality. In his typology of biologic, religious, creative, and natural symbolic ways we "live on" beyond our deaths, our artificial selves represent a blend of creative and simulated biology. Will carebots lead us to more trustingly acknowledge the unparalleled worth of our instruments as wings of progress, our inheritance from Daedalus? Or, bearing the hubris of Icarus, will we trust our wings blindly as a means to self-aggrandizement? Will we become heirs to Daedalus' talent and perspective, or to Icarus' conceit? Or both? Human hubris, so evidently depicted in Icarus' flight and fall, against his father Daedalus' warnings about getting too close to both the sun and sea, remains the perennial conductor of our runaway train. The threat lies not with robots. In lies in how we humans view them and interact with them, and, moreover, how we think of ourselves and our relation with other humans.

NOTES

1. David Hochman, "18 Weeks," *AARP Bulletin* 61, no. 10 (December 2020): 8.
2. Dana-Claudia Thompson, Madalina-Gabriela Barbu, Cristina Beiu, Lilliana Gabriela Popa, Mara Madalina Mihai, Mihai Berteanu, and Marius Nicolae Popescu, "The Impact of COVID-19 Pandemic on Long-Term Care Facilities Worldwide:

An Overview on International Issues," *BioMed Research International*, Article ID 8870249 (November 11, 2020): 2, 4–5, https://doi.org/10.1155/2020/8870249.

3. Hochman, "18 Weeks," 16.

4. Hochman, "18 Weeks," 12.

5. Amisha Parekh de Campos and Susan Daniels, "Ethical Implications of COVID-19: Palliative Care, Public Health, and Long-Term Care Facilities," *Journal of Hospice and Palliative Nursing* 23, no. 2 (April 2021): 120–127.

6. M. Keith Chen, Judith A. Chevalier, and Elisa F. Long, "Nursing Home Staff Networks and COVID-19," *PNAS, Proceedings of the National Academy of Sciences of the United States of America* 118, no. 1 (Jan. 5, 2021): 3, https://doi.org/10.1073/pnas.2015455118.

7. Chen et al., "Nursing Home Staff Networks," 1.

8. Chen et al., "Nursing Home Staff Networks," 1.

9. Hochman, "18 Weeks," 14.

10. Hochman, "18 Weeks," 14.

11. Joe Eaton, "Who Is to Blame," *AARP Bulletin* 61, no. 10 (December 2020): 23.

12. Hochman, "18 Weeks," 12.

13. Shannon Vallor, "Carebots and Caregivers: Sustaining the Ethical Ideal of Xare in the 21st Century," *Journal of Philosophy and Technology* 24 (2011): 251–68.

14. Eric Topol, *Deep Medicine: How Artificial Intelligence Can Make Healthcare Human Again* (New York: Basic Books, 2019), 54–55.

15. Topol, *Deep Medicine*, 55.

16. Topol, *Deep Medicine*, 61–64.

17. Kazuo Ishiguro, *Klara and the Sun* (New York: Alfred A. Knopf, 2021).

18. Ishiguro, *Klara and the Sun*, 26.

19. S. Kay Toombs, "The Role of Empathy in Clinical Practice," in *Between Ourselves: Second-Person Issues in the Study of Consciousness*, ed. Evan Thompson (Thorverton, U.K.: Imprint Academic, 2001), 257.

20. Michael B. A. Oldstone, *Viruses, Plagues, and History* (New York: Oxford University Press, 1998), 186.

21. David Quammen, *Spillover: Animal Infections and the Next Human Pandemic* (New York: W.W. Norton & Company, 2012), 20.

22. Victoria Gill, "Coronavirus: This Is Not the Last Pandemic," BBC News, June 6, 2020, https://www.bbc.com/news/science-environment-52775386.

23. Michael T. Osterholm and Mark Olshaker, *Deadliest Enemy: Our War against Killer Germs* (New York Little, Brown Spark, 2017), 263.

24. Osterholm and Olshaker, *Deadliest Enemy*, 264.

25. Osterholm and Olshaker, *Deadliest Enemy*, 264.

26. Andrew Hawkins, "The world's first robot car death was the result of human error—and it can happen again," *The Verge*, Nov. 20, 2019, https://www.theverge.com/2019/11/20/20973971/uber-self-driving-car-crash-investigation-human-error-results.

27. Cited in *AI in Healthcare*, Summer 2018, 6, https://www.purestorage.com/content/dam/pdf/en/thought-leadership/protected/tl-ai-in-healthcare-article.pdf.

28. John Cohen, *Human Robots in Myth and Science* (London: Allen and Unwin, 1966), 137.

Chapter One

Are Robots Made for This?

The divine blacksmith Hephaestus has been busy. Commissioned by Zeus on behalf of his son Minos, King of Crete, Hephaestus created the giant bronze guardian Talos, humanlike in form. Talos was our first robot. His mission: to routinely patrol the island of Crete and guard against invaders, whom he would immediately destroy by hurling huge boulders at incoming vessels. He would press survivors to his red-hot chest and burn them alive. Under the threat of invasion, he was made for this, to protect. Our mythic Coast Guard with its motto, semper paratus, always ready.

Our first robot, however, was also mortal. The sorceress Medea knew this. She knew Talos' weak spot, his Achilles Heel, a bolt located at his ankle sealing in his life-fluid, ichor. Without ichor, Talos was useless. In his epic poem, Argonautica, Appolonius of Rhodes tells us that Jason and his Argonauts, facing dead wind, sheltered their ship Argo by Crete's steep cliffs. Talos immediately spotted them and, as programmed, began hurling rocks at the ship. The cunning Medea comes to the aid of the Argonauts and bewitches Talos so that, disoriented, he stumbles against a sharp rock that pierces his ankle, loosening the bolt. The giant guardian then crumbles as his life-force, his ichor, flows out of him. Medea knew her opponent.[1]

Our visions of the promise of artificial life run deep. As ancient myths depict, we have long yearned to create our own beings. These myths unmask indelible truths about us, here, now, and always. The relationship between myth and science is no closed door. Legends and tales of gods creating artificial life confirm their inexorable kinship. These tales form the nucleus of a culture's worldview related through symbols and a timeless narrative. Myths house stories of some long-ago that unveil hidden plots of our present. Paul Ricoeur writes that "myth relates to the events that happened at the beginning of time which have the purpose of providing grounds for the ritual actions of men today."[2] Mythic narrative is a mingling of selective remembrance, real-time discernment, and anticipation of what will come In essence, myths fuse creative origins and likely eschatologies.

The giant guardian Talos is human in resemblance. When a creation like Talos is made to appear more similar in form and behavior to human beings, its creature status changes to a "being." And the notion of a "being" "made, not born" goes beyond the figurative. Our life-long relationship with our creations bears this out. Hegel's dialectic of history annuls time's linearity and exposes its circle of what was, is, and will be. As for myth, Paul Ricoeur's "mythic time" is a "third form of time" distinct from human and cosmic history. Mythic time precedes the human historic narrative. Mythic time, the tales we refer to in this book at the start of our chapters, "embraces the totality of what we designate as, on the one hand, the world and, on the other hand, human existence."[3] In short, myth recalls this "great time" that enfolds time's totality, placing our microscopic human history within the perspective of "cosmic time." Ricoeur writes, "This mythic time, far from plunging thought into a night where all cows are black, initiates a unique, overall scansion, by ordering in terms of one another cycles of different duration, the great celestial cycles, biological recurrences, and the rhythms of social life."[4]

HUMAN AND MACHINE: AN OLD DANCE

When it comes to our "rhythms of social life," interacting with machines is hardly new. Every time we email, text, tweet, research online, ask 'Siri' or 'Alexa' questions ("Siri, how far is it from Cardiff, Wales to Cambridge, England?"), even talk to our cars, iPhones, TVs, and teddy bears, we are 'connecting' with and through a nonliving object. Many of us have our own Linus blanket of security—some good luck charm, token, special coffee mug, rosary, photo, cap, tennis socks (athletes are notorious for their good luck tokens and rituals), beliefs, superstitions, and habits. Even though St. Christopher had been deposed from the official army of Catholic saints, and because Christopher is my Confirmation name, I travel with my St. Christopher medal.

When it comes to healthcare, our interfacing with machines is a given, particularly now in our digital universe in which digital technologies have permeated nearly every corner of our lives, from home to higher-education, banking, airlines, countless consumer goods, etc. Since the introduction of computerized records, the spawning of electronic medical records (EMR, or electronic health records, EHR) has led to the ubiquitous presence of computers and laptops throughout healthcare settings. We will discuss this further in chapter 3. For now, this human-machine interaction, while offering numerous advantages over the older, error-prone system, turns out to be a shaky marriage, and medical mistakes persist. In the spirit of psychiatrist Ronald Heifetz's classic distinction between technical problems and adaptive problems in the context of institutional leadership, many of the problems we face with new technologies are not due to the technologies themselves, but are adaptive, having to do with human attitude, adaptation, and learning about the technologies. In contrast, technical problems are mechanical in nature, addressed by fixing the tools.[5] So, it comes as no surprise that, just as medical specialties like gastroenterology and cardiology have their own strict requirements and board certifications, the new and growing specialty of medical informatics intends to help ease that troubling relation we humans have with our technologies.

However, as we have come to realize throughout our long COVID blight, despite the wonders and comfort our machines and devices offer, they are not the same as the touch and embrace we get from a living, flesh and blood being, human or non-human animal. Connectivity via objects and devices is not the same as human-to-human connectedness. How we have interacted with each other during our plague is proof. Without doubt, our digital communicative technologies are invaluable and life-saving. But, again, *connectivity is not connectedness*. Genuine connectedness demands physical, embodied interaction and presence. This brings us to the question we address in this book. Can we have this kind of connectedness with a caring robot? Or is the caring that carebots offer counterfeit? Are we ready at this point to make the claim that carebot-caring is fake and human-caring is real? Remember that Talos, our first bot, was created to protect the inhabitants of the island of Crete. Myths about artificial life spark us to reflect on our human-artifice interaction. Will our interaction with our creations give birth to some mutation in how we communicate, how we see, think of, and relate to other humans? And the more barbed test—will it affect how we think of ourselves?

A New Bot Partner: Carebots

Let us first be cautious of lumping together "robots." There are many kinds of robots along with varied areas of robotic applications such as in epigenetic, cognitive, affective, and rehabilitative robotics with distinct purposes and functions.[6] There are those autonomous robots appearing more frequently in Korean and Japanese shopping malls as guides and self-standing information centers. The social robots now being designed as companions and assistants are different from robots' origins. The term "robot," from the Czech *robota* meaning "servitude" or "drudgery," was first used in Karel Čapek's written 1920 play "R.U.R.," "Rossum's Universal Robots." Performed the following year, his play depicts a future scenario when artificial humans, called *robota*, are mass-produced as laborers. Čapek's *robota*, made from protoplasmic goo, not metal and wires, are indistinguishable in appearance from humans and lack ethnic differences.

His newer models of *robota* were designed with emotions, and they end up revolting against humans and killing them all except one. Bear in mind, the performance of "R.U.R." occurred in the aftermath of worker revolts in Hungary, Germany, and Russia. The rebellion of robots shows how human interaction with robots mirrors how we treat other humans, particularly in relations of power and authority.

The tale is strikingly prescient of Philip K. Dick's 1968 classic *Do Androids Dream of Electric Sheep?* The film version "Blade Runner," though a classic, falls radically short of the book. No surprise there. The book demands more from the reader. Yet in both the book and film, replicants are only distinguished from humans by their level of empathy, indicated by the dilation of their pupils in response to situations of threat, pain, and suffering. Replicants are bio-engineered to work on space colonies. After a handful escape and land on earth, a bounty hunter seeks them out to "retire" them. The key lesson in "R.U.R." and *Do Androids Dream of Electric Sheep?* captures what we stress throughout our chapters: Our interface with robots reveals much about us.

Take Japan. The Japanese have carved out a somewhat comfortable rapport with robots as service assistants, companions, friends, even heroes. The culture's *zeitgeist* toward technology holds an optimistic view concerning a symbiotic bond between humans and robots, the latter often exemplifying how we humans can overcome our hurdles. Technology is not considered as some Other in an antagonist, oppressive, threateningly ambiguous relationship, a dystopic perspective we find more widespread in the West as evident in box-office hits like "Blade Runner," "Matrix," "Blade Runner 2049," "A.I. Artificial Intelligence," "Ghost in the Shell," "Minority Report," "Ex Machina," and the British TV series "Humans." In contrast, Astro Boy, Japan's long-popular and beloved robot in *manga* (comics), is almost human, a trusting friend with superpowers, but his human-likeness comes with the usual bundle of human doubts, vulnerabilities, and fears. Astro Boy is unique, not like other robots. He has a spirit, *kami*, as does all of nature, natural forces, and living beings, and he works autonomously, as moral agent, for the good of others. His affinity, or humanlikeness, makes him all the more appealing. He is a role model for humans, demonstrating the possibility that we too can overcome our inner demons and work for the welfare of others.

At the same time, the power of robots has its dark side. How we have adapted to communicating with each other during our long pandemic attests to the longstanding relation we have had with devices. They influence us in more ways than we think. For instance, bots have been rather active in the Twitter universe churning out information about the nature of the virus. We may presume that reliable humans are informing us about the disease, alleged cures, and encouraging the reopening of businesses and schools and resisting any restrictive directives. However, analysts have made the gritty discovery that countless tweets from these 'experts' have come from bots. This bot activity, surmised to be orchestrated by Russian or Chinese 'agents' has spurred all sorts of irrational, paranoiac, poisonous conspiracy theories lights years from solid science and common sense.[7]

Back in 2011, when caring robots like GeckoSystems' CareBot™ for elders were first appearing on the market, I wrote a futuristic twist on this theme about my hospice robot, Seamus.[8] Perhaps it was farfetched then, but it is more likely now, a time soon to come when we will have caring robots, even for hospice care, customized to suit our needs. Seamus was responsive to my expressions and feelings, and, most importantly, always attentive. 'He' faithfully wrote down notes I dictated for my final book and, like my Dad, always had a joke. Seamus was easy to be with. He dutifully monitored my vital signs, pulse, blood pressure, and heart rate, and remained ready to alert Brooke or 911 when necessary. Whenever I missed my medications, Seamus would never fail to remind me. He was, like Talos for Cretans, my own personal lifeguard. Carebots like Seamus promise to become an invaluable commodity in the near future for the following practical reasons. Our dramatic global demographic upsurge of seniors needing more care at home means an intensifying demand for caregivers. Compared to human caregivers, carebots are low-cost and without the need for health benefits. They are also accommodating, supportive, efficient, and reliable. Moreover, not only are carebots free from typical family entanglements, but, more importantly, they provide relief for families and human caregivers. In circumstances of contagion, they can save lives. In future pandemics, with carebots in long-term care settings, nursing homes will no longer be the plague's epicenter. Personally, with Seamus looking after me, I can feel wanted. Cared for.

Whether Seamus genuinely *cares for* me is another matter. Philosopher Nel Noddings tells us that caring is life's most primal drive, a fundamental moral disposition. She writes

> Caring involves stepping outside of one's personal frame of reference into the other's. When we care, we consider the other's point of view, his objective needs, and what he expects of us. Our attention, our mental engrossment is on the cared-for, not on ourselves. Our reasons for acting, then, have to do both with the other's wants and desires and with the objective elements of his problematic situation.[9]

Can Seamus step *outside* of his own frame of reference? Does he even have one? If so, does he have the will to do so and choose to care for me? He may perform selflessly. But does he have a "self" to transcend? For sure, Seamus *acts* reliably. But this is different from *being* reliable. The honor behind dependability lies in the fact that it is our choice: we choose to be dependable, or not. Although Seamus is a "companion" who at least *performs* acts of caregiving, when I someday face the Void, if Seamus is there, will that make a difference?[10]

COVID'S TOLL ON HEALTHCARE WORKERS

Can we have a genuine relationship, a connectedness, with a caring robot? Like my hospice robot Seamus, their instrumental value is without doubt. And in view of the surging global demographics of seniors and the never-ending need for caregivers, along with carebots' cost-savings, efficiency, reliability, around-the-clock accessibility, performative and life-saving support, we cannot dispute their worth particularly during times of contagion. Without question, they can help ease the terrible drain on our healthcare workers and families. Looking at their burden with a wide lens can offer a glimpse of how carebots in the future can save lives and relieve anguish.

The toll of this pandemic on healthcare workers has been crushing, exacting alarming shortages of healthcare professionals and equally disturbing levels of moral distress. Because of fears of infection, schools had shut down forcing education to occur at home where most working parents must either stay and work from there or go to their work site if necessary. Many healthcare workers and first responders, urgently needed in hospitals, clinics, and emergency units, are working parents. But they also need to be with their children to help them navigate Zoom, Webex, or other 'learning' labyrinths. The dire shortage of healthcare and emergency providers that we faced can be alleviated by the 24/7 availability of carebots. Though carebots cannot address the untold human angst, they can at least help alleviate the crushing weight our healthcare workers carry. They can monitor and test patients without complaint, fatigue, health benefits, and without the moral aches providers have experienced tenfold. Without doubt, healthcare workers who have cared for the potentially and already infected patients suffer terribly high levels of stress, a strain that does end with their work shift. And the stress mounts when there is little in the way of institutional support. Add to that the frequent media accounts we heard of nurses, practitioners, and other professionals not having enough personal protective equipment, being instructed to re-use their N95 masks, compelled to cut trash bags for further protection, clearly in the trenches without enough weapons. Such stories have been amplified incessantly through the echo-chamber of a mainstream media that needs to be held morally accountable for stirring national fear, anxiety, and despair.

Agonizing accounts give evidence for the benefits of having carebots take the place of human caregivers during these sorts of crises. Barbara

Birchenough was a 65-year-old nurse at Clara Maass Medical Center in Belleville, New Jersey. After a safety complaint was issued about the hospital's policies, even though the veteran Birchenbough was not working directly with COVID patients, some patients under her care showed COVID symptoms. Barbara contracted the disease and died within weeks. That same day, her co-worker, 62-year-old veteran nursing aide Nestor Bautista, also died of COVID-19. During Barbara's agonizing shift at the medical center, she sent a text to her daughter: "The ICU nurses are making gowns out of garbage bags. Dad is going to pick up large garbage bags for me just in case." She later began to show symptoms and texted, "Please pray for all health care workers, we are running out of supplies."[11]

When Brandon Rogers, after beating cancer asked his friend Vincent DeJesus if he would go with him to get his medical test results, Vincent sent him a text: "I can't. I got the COVID . . . I'm sorry bro but I wish you luck. You got this."[12] That gives a sense of Vincent's selflessness, thinking of others first, like making sure he did not infect his 69-year-old mother, a former nurse, who lived with him. DeJesus, a 39-year-old nurse who worked at Sunrise Hospital and Medical Center in Las Vegas, died of COVID-19 after working with COVID patients, convinced that his surgical mask and face shield probably would not be enough to protect him. He was right. Nurses unions demanded that Gov. Sisolak and the Occupational Safety and Health Administration (OSHA) mandate safety standards above the Centers for Disease Control and Prevention (CDC) minimum. This was in August 2020.[13] Over 4,000 safety complaints regarding lack of protective equipment swamped various states' OSHA offices with little in the way of OSHA follow-up while deaths among healthcare workers continued to mount.[14] Not having enough personal protective equipment, healthcare workers were handcuffed. In some cases they were also threatened with institutional retaliation or termination if they publicly complained. Kaiser Health News reporters wrote in their June 2020 account:

> Of the 4,100-plus complaints that flooded OSHA offices, over two-thirds are now marked as "closed" in an OSHA database. Among them was a complaint that staffers handling dead bodies in a small room off the lobby of a Manhattan nursing home weren't given appropriate protective gear. More than 100 of those cases were resolved within 10 days. One of those complaints said home health nurses in the Bronx were sent to treat COVID-19 patients without full protective gear. At a Massachusetts nursing home that housed COVID patients, staff members were asked to wash and reuse masks and disposable gloves, another complaint said.[15]

The U.S. touts itself as the world's best in medical care. However, a 2019 Commonwealth Fund study tells a different story.[16] It compared the U.S. health system to ten other high-income countries—Australia, Canada, France, Germany, the Netherlands, New Zealand, Norway, Sweden, Switzerland, and the United Kingdom—using data from the Organization for Economic Co-operation and Development (OECD). The study also compared the U.S. to the OECD average, comprising thirty-six member countries. Here are the findings. We still have low life expectancy, high suicide rates, exceptionally higher levels of chronic disease and obesity, less frequent physician visits, overuse of expensive technologies, the most hospitalizations from preventable causes, and the highest rate of avoidable deaths. One silver lining is that we outperform our peers when it comes to breast cancer screenings and flu vaccinations for those 65 and older. However, given that the U.S. spends more than any other country on healthcare, the health return on investment is far from superior. It is therefore not surprising that when COVID-19 appeared in the US and mushroomed within weeks, we were clearly ill-prepared. And with the government sidestepping critical considerations, an already overtaxed healthcare system faced its set of Sisyphean challenges. Healthcare workers, not only in hospitals but particularly in residential facilities, outpatient clinics, hospices, and prisons daily faced a life-and-death gauntlet due to insufficient and inequitable access to testing, a nationwide scarcity of protective equipment, resistance and politicization of common sense measures such as physical distancing and mask-wearing, and a good deal of public unawareness and denial of the magnitude of the real threat of the contagion. Clearly, the supply chain crisis and not enough N95s helped to peak angst among healthcare workers, particularly nurses and physicians on the front lines. At the start, it was believed that the typical surgical mask, along with a face shield, would be safe enough for those caring for COVID patients. However, bear in mind that the earlier CDC guidelines were formed on the basis of the 2003 SARS outbreak. It did not take long to realize that COVID-19 was a different airborne beast, one that was asymptomatic.

Global Misery

The global plight thickens the misery soup. COVID-19 has claimed well over 4 million lives.[17] According to a joint study by Amnesty International, Public Services International (PSI), and UNI Global Union, as of March 2021, the global number of deaths included over 17,000 healthcare workers.[18] These include nurses, nurse practitioners, aides, physicians, assistants, orderlies, technicians, staff, volunteers, administrators, drivers, porters, etc., employed and retired. The report stressed the urgent need for fair vaccine access and distribution for all frontline healthcare workers. The pandemic has clearly opened many of the cracks in health systems and governments worldwide. One gaping fissure is the scandalous disparities in vaccine access between rich and poor countries. The study asserts that, at the time it was published, "More than half the world's doses have so far been administered in just 10 rich countries, making up less than 10 percent of the world's population, while over 100 countries are yet to vaccinate a single person."[19] The unsafe environment and dire shortages of personal protective equipment that American healthcare workers faced has magnified in countries like Mexico, Brazil, Malaysia, Peru, South Africa, and now India. Further factors such as thin and inconsistent supply chains and distribution, along with questions as to who counts as a "healthcare worker" plainly add to the burden. Cleaners, sanitation groups, and social workers should count as frontline workers along with nursing home workers and home care assistants. Yet they are often overlooked and their crucial work is minimized. As Steve Cockburn, Amnesty International's Head of Economic and Social Justice, states "For one health worker to die from COVID-19 every 30 minutes is both a tragedy and an injustice ... Urgent action must be taken to close the huge global inequalities in vaccine access, so that a community health worker in Peru is protected as much as a doctor in the UK."[20] Globally, this lack of access and absence of personal protective equipment has exacted a jarring toll on healthcare workers. Imagine what they faced. Envision being summoned to work with possibly infectious patients without sufficient protection, knowing that once we leave the hospital we put our families and others at risk.

In the U.S., because the government in the last administration poorly tracked healthcare worker fatalities, leaving the tracking to individual hospitals and private sectors, conflicting reports have impaired any accurate count.[21] "Lost on the Frontline," a year-long investigation by *The Guardian* and Kaiser Health News, reported 3,607 U.S. healthcare workers lives lost in the pandemic's first year. That amounts to almost 2,000 more than reported by the CDC. The report's findings revealed the following: half of the deaths were of those under 60 years of age; the majority were identified as persons of color; most of the deaths were of nurses and support staff; most victims worked in the five hardest hit states of New York, Texas, California, New Jersey, and Florida; most victims worked in residential facilities, outpatient clinics, and hospices and prisons with 25 percent working at hospitals.[22] This "Lost on the Frontline" project involved over 100 reporters. Not only does it offer detailed information and statistics, but includes victims' faces and their stories. This is imperative. Faces showing personhood and singularity emasculate cold statistics. They bear witness to the unspeakable loss in many cases aggravated by the dire lack of N95 masks and personal protective equipment.

Social Calamity

Innumerable accounts of the tragic, lonely deaths of COVID-19 victims prove the virus' social collateral damage, particularly the ban against being there in-person with patients during their final weeks, days, and hours. Because family were not allowed in a patient's room and even the hospital, a nurse at the bedside often held an iPhone or tablet up to the patient for one last Facetime visit with a spouse, child, sibling, or other family member. One of the dreaded fears dying patients have is that of being alone with no one to simply *be there*. Luke Fildes' remarkable painting, "The Doctor," remains a testimony to this being-there, this presence.[23] It depicts the family doctor at a time, 1891, without antibiotics and remedy from the raging disease then, tuberculosis. The painter and his wife are in the shadowy background as the doctor sits by the bed of their little girl dying from the disease. The doctor can offer no cure. That came in 1944 with streptomycin. But in late Victorian London, all he can do is be with the little girl and stay there, until the end. Many times the real patient(s) is not the patient. And being there, for the distressed parents, can make all the difference.

Ironically, with new treatments, this being-there, presence, has lost its currency. Today, we have cures for all types of disease. It is a marvelous time of medical breakthroughs. But the scourge of COVID-19 has been a different beast, and being there in-person with the patient is not viable. Consider the hundreds of ultra-Orthodox Jews who have died in Brooklyn, New York, particularly in the Crown Heights area. Says neighborhood Hasidic rabbi Avraham Berkowitz, "that whole religious power of comfort, that is gone. They're locked alone with a video camera. I had to do Zoom shiva calls."[24] Because families are not permitted to be with their loved ones in their final days at Borough Park's Maimonides Medical Center, Director of Operations of the Chesed Shel Emes Burial Society Mayer Berger established a hotline with prerecorded Jewish prayers. As Berger describes, "People can have a patient rep in a hospital calling the hotline, and put the prayers on speaker right next to the people who passed away."[25]

We took part in drive-by funerals with mourners in cars as we watched the casket lowered into the earth by funeral home staff wearing masks and gloves. Being there to embrace each other is not feasible when the best expression of caring for a loved one comes with keeping our distance. As restrictions prohibited public wakes and funerals, family members grieved alone. Though online condolences poured in, what was missing was the physical presence of friends together at a time when being there in-person means everything. For each person who dies, several survivors remain at risk. They risk grieving without healing and moving on. In some respects, closure is a myth. It is too tidy. Matters of the heart are always left unfinished. But at least grieving properly is crucial. Without it, problems creep in, physical and emotional, like sleep disruption, increased blood pressure, drug and alcohol dependency, ulcerative colitis, depression, suicidality, and interpersonal dysfunction. The embodied presence of others who share our grief gives us strength, and empowers us to re-enter life's stream, though now radically altered from our loss. Mourning together with others in-the-flesh is a whisper of the divine in our midst. And although cards and online condolences offer a safe substitute, they can never replace genuine face-to-face presence, being there together. As we will discuss in chapter 4, the face speaks its own language, beyond words. It is our conduit for engagement with each other. The face is an epiphany that ruptures our routine immersion in our online world. The face also reminds us that statistics and numbers never really measure suffering. For us survivors, how we regret missing that last chance to say goodbye and to tell them that we love them.[26]

The presence of carebots in the future will not erase much of this tragedy when we face other, looming pandemics. Nonetheless, they can emphatically ease the yoke on healthcare workers and caregivers worldwide. And with carebots lessening the care-taking burden, human caregivers can be freer to interact face-to-face with the cared-for, to engage with them more personally so that their last days and moments are not alone. This in turn helps relieve the anguish of family members who helplessly stand by and watch as their loved ones die, for their loved one will not be alone. Carebots seem to be made for these sorts of crises: to monitor, support, and provide care in so many useful and life-saving ways. This brings us back to the scope and nature of caregiving that we can expect from carebots in the near future. Again, can a carebot replace a human caregiver?

TEACH ME TO REPLACE YOU

Each question begets another, and another, etc. That is the threatening beauty of philosophy. We are always in deep water when we philosophize. The question—can we have a real relationship with a caring robot?—arouses the further question of whether carebots themselves can really care. What kind of caring can they offer? Is it a matter of substance or degree? Have we boosted the skills in AI enough for the machine with its algorithmic brain to ask us, point-blank, Can you teach me to replace you? Not as your occasional substitute or stand-in, but to act, perform, respond, interact just like you. To *be* you. The question plainly puzzles us humans. After all, we start with unspoken metaphysical and epistemic rules. One such tenet is that when it comes to caring, no matter how you cut it, robots are incapable of caring because they are incapable of feeling, and that is because they lack a mind of their own.

The deeper silent dogma, our human conceit, is that we are each individually irreplaceable. Yet when we pose that question in the context of a non-alive material object of our own making, the question takes on new meaning. This leads us to the entrenched challenge in artificial intelligence—replicating human processes, particularly human thinking.

Our ever-fluid human-machine gestalt compels us for now to put aside the age-old philosophical conundrum of 'mind' and its conventional propositions regarding the relation between mind and brain. At the same time, we cannot ignore those established mind-brain theories ranging from mind-brain identity, to the epiphenomenalist distinction without a difference, to the outright dualist notion that the mind and brain remain separable, a notion less fashionable these days. Instead, let us start with a clear-headed, key presupposition: while we are alive, our mental life is inextricably somehow wrapped up with our brain life. That is all that matters at this point. No surprise that AI is not concerned with the Hereafter, whatever versions we give it. It is about the Here Now. The question irreducibly pares down to this: In view of our mind's natural intercourse with the brain, can we replicate the human brain? Philip K. Dick's title, *Do Androids Dream of Electric Sheep?* nicely captures the challenge as does his novel, much better than Ridley Scott's 1982 film noir "Blade Runner" that only loosely unpacks the novel's philosophical currency and real question, Can we replicate the human brain? Denis Villeneuve's 2017 "Blade Runner 2049" tunnels deeper into the existential grotto and responds: When androids dream, they dream of becoming human. This is evident in the film's centerpiece, the biological 'miracle' of the replicant Rachael (from the original film) having given birth to a baby girl and boy while herself dying in childbirth. This further stirs the pot vis-à-vis actually replicating the human brain.

The Riddle

Tough riddles are fine-tuned to test our brain power. Consider medical diagnosis, an intricate, complex process that can be stubbornly shaded with varying degrees of uncertainty that is part of the medical drama. The late distinguished medical sociologist and my dear friend Renée C. Fox studied and wrote eloquently about medical uncertainty. From her experience and research on Boston's Peter Bent Brigham Hospital's Ward F-Second, and influenced by her mentor and noted sociologist Talcott Parsons, she conducted first-hand, face-to-face interaction with patients and physicians that resulted in her classic *Experiment Perilous*, an account of physicians facing the stress of having to come to terms with their dual mission of caring for their patients while at the same time conducting experimental clinical research having uncertain results. At that time, Ward F-Second was the hospital's eminent research ward for patients most of whom were terminally ill. A number of them had prostate cancer and malignant hypertension.[27] From her work, she proposed three basic kinds of uncertainty. Two involved the 1) human inability to capture the vast scope of medical knowledge and 2) recognizing significant gaps and limits to this overwhelmingly vast corpus of knowledge. The Socratic equation: the more we know, the more we do not know, and wisdom lies in knowing the difference. 3) The third type of uncertainty deals with the challenges physicians and particularly medical students face in discerning the quality of what they do know, or better, what they think they know.

> The first results from incomplete or imperfect mastery of available knowledge. No one can have at his command all skills and all knowledge of the lore of medicine. The second depends upon limitations in current medical knowledge. There are innumerable questions to which no physician, however well trained, can as yet provide answers. A third source of uncertainty derives from the first two. This consists of difficulty in distinguishing between personal ignorance or ineptitude and the limitations of present medical knowledge.[28]

In their *The Courage to Fail* where they tackle the ever-thorny issues in organ transplantation, she and Judith Swazey write about the inexorable quandaries surrounding medical uncertainty.

> Our formulation of the problems of uncertainty that transplantation and dialysis entail progressively came to include phenomena as diverse as the biological mysteries of the rejection reaction, the ambiguities of the relationship between clinical experimentation and therapy . . . problematic aspects of clinical moratorium, and the dilemmas involved in allocating various kinds of scarce resources.[29]

In her later narrative biography, *In the Field*, Fox reaffirms the need for physicians and students to come to terms with the daunting challenge medical uncertainty presents, alluding to her invaluable experience working with doctors and patients on Ward F-Second.

> I was highly attuned to issues of medical uncertainty by the time that I had spent in the midst of the physicians and patients of Ward F-Second . . . But there is cogent evidence, independent of the resonance that it already had for me, that training for uncertainty is considered by medical educators and students alike to be one of the most crucial and challenging aspects of the process of becoming a physician . . . despite all the changes in medical knowledge, and the recurring reforms in medical school curricula that have occurred during the ensuing fifty years, medical students still give spontaneous testimony to the exceptional importance of learning to recognize that "medicine is filled with uncertainty,"

and to deal psychologically, as well as cognitively, with the implications of this inevitable fact for the care of their future patients.[30]

If we take the routine differential diagnosis that culls together the facts, relevant symptoms and signs, weighs tests, assigns various hypotheses, rules some out and keeps others in, piecing together and connecting the dots, paying more attention to some (e.g., the patient's home lifestyle, exercise habits, diet, stress, and sleep) than to others, and arrive at the most probable explanation, medical diagnosis is high-stakes detective work. One that goes from hypothesis to appropriate treatment, the results of which can either confirm the diagnosis or rule it out. As a simple example, during this pandemic if I lived reclusively for months in an isolated cabin deep in the woods of Maine, going out well-masked only for medical appointments and essential grocery visits to nearby Belfast, and get tested regarding infection, I am highly unlikely to have the virus. So when my test results come back positive, there is good reason to test again. If, after another test, I am again tested positive as having the virus, we rightly wonder how. Medical diagnosis, an immensely complex process the late surgeon Sherwin Nuland called "The Riddle," forms the essential knowledge-based empirical cornerstone of what it means to be a physician.[31] Nuland writes:

> The quest of every doctor in approaching serious disease is to make the diagnosis and to design and carry out the specific cure. This quest I call The Riddle, and I capitalize it so there will not be mistaking its dominance over every other consideration. The satisfaction of solving The Riddle is its own reward, and the fuel that drives the clinical engines of medicine's most highly trained specialists. It is every doctor's measure of his own abilities; it is the most important ingredient in his professional self-image.[32]

This delivers the point-blank challenge for AI in medicine. Can AI match this skill, this art? This medical cornerstone forms the basis for a physician's art in curing, alleviating morbidity, in caring and healing. The two pillars of healing and caring are less knowledge-derived, but come from empathy. Whether AI can replicate human empathy is another, plucky question that we will later address.

Extended Mind

For now, let us stay on track with the challenge AI research tenaciously tackles in replicating human cognition. In effect, our human-machine interface is a type of 'social' interacting in the spirit of Bruno Latour's 'assemblages' of how we relate to our tools, like the uniquely personal relation I have with the pen that initially writes all this on paper as well as my relation with the computer keyboard that now relays these words and ideas on to software.³³ Latour's notion is reminiscent of philosophers Andy Clark and David Chalmers' theory of the extended mind.³⁴ They pose their theory to challenge the longstanding conventional view, inherited in many respects from Descartes though foreshadowed much earlier, of mind, or mental activity, being seated in the brain. This orthodox view holds that mind is intimately private. It is my mind and not yours, inevitably conjuring the quandary of whether I can know your mind. For Clark and Chalmers, their view of mind as extended is not merely a metaphor in that my pen and keyboard simply *express* what I am thinking. In contrast, mind is literally extended in space. They illustrate this idea with their classic example of Inga and Otto. Suffering from early Alzheimer's Disease, Otto relies on his address book for directions. Inga's memory is perfectly fine. They both wish to attend the recent exhibit at New York's Museum of Modern Art. Whereas Otto in the past would have known how to get there from memory, he now depends upon his address book. Inga, on the other hand, with her normal recall has no need for an address book. According to Clark and Chalmers, Otto literally extends his mind to his address book. The address book has become, spatially, a part of Otto's mind.³⁵ In similar fashion, the notebook in which I write tangibly manifests my mind, extended beyond my body. Although my notebook, housing my inscribed thoughts on its pages, is materially outside my brain, it also physically manifests this 'mind' that I think of as mine. As private as I believe my mind is, it is not confined within my skull. Hence, Clark claims we are all "natural cyborgs."³⁶

Clark and Chalmers offer a persuasive and no doubt influential argument, though not beyond dispute. On what ground can I assert that my notebook is in effect literally *similar* to my thoughts while writing? Is there any physical, tangible continuity? Philosophers Paul Dumouchel and Luisa Damiano raise this challenge and propose that any "physical unity" between a material object and mind does not exist. Instead, they suggest a "mental relation" or "relation of signification." For them, rather than "extended," the mind is "distributed."³⁷ Their claim makes sense since Clark and Chalmers' rather materialist thesis is one in which their "extended mind" remains seated in an individual brain, and this primary residency in the brain still affirms a Cartesian dominion of an "I" housed in my body. In other words, as Dumouchel and Damiano assert, we conventionally think of cognition and mentation, or mental activity, modeled upon our limited human construct. They fittingly cite philosopher Paul Humphreys' contention that this established assumption still glues us to an "anthropocentrism" in how we consider "mind." Humphreys aptly reminds us of how our advanced technologies and machines unmistakably outperform humans in scope, efficiency, and speed.³⁸ Machine cognition such as genetic coding, IBM's Watson for Health, tabulating financial input and stocks, etc. easily surpasses human cognition. The machine's deep cognitive bowels are far beyond human comprehension, giving us little ground to hang on to the Protagorean notion that we are the "measure of all things."

Nonetheless, we still cling to any vestige of human hegemony. Are we not the ones who interpret and make sense of the data? We are still the ones who *know* and *understand*. But just how much authority do we really have? Dumouchel and Damiano's example of the U.S. Patriot Air and Missile Defense System is apropos. Its AI system's cognitive plus intuitive aptitude fluently performs the knowing and interpreting processes. It recognizes a real threat and responds accordingly through trajectory calculations and sets up a launch. Yet human operators can still intervene and abort. Strong counterpoint. But while Dumouchel and Damiano underscore the defense system's cognitive autonomy they also alert us to the fact that mistakes are not the same as mechanical errors. That is, precisely *because* the system is cognitive, it is capable of making mistakes.

> Surely it would be exceedingly odd to say that this system is cognitive only when a human being supervises its operation. The very fact that we depend upon a human being to supervise the system suggests that we are indeed dealing with a cognitive system. The human operator is there to guard against the chance that the system "makes a mistake." Mind you, only cognitive systems make mistakes; mechanical systems break down—but they do not make mistakes![39]

In other words, cognition, that aspect of the all-encompassing and yet innately vague umbrella "mind," may well exist *outside* of our heads. There is the human mind, and there is a farther-reaching "cognitive domain." To insist that cognition does not go beyond our bodies reflects our human epistemic hubris.

> The existence of so vast and varied a network testifies to exactly this, the heterogeneity of the cognitive domain, within which human beings constitute a cognitive system of a particular type, but one that is neither the only possible cognitive system nor the most perfectly cognitive system, much less the indisputable criterion of what counts as cognition.[40]

In a sense their "ecology of mind" reflects the Buddhist *pratityasamutpada*, or "rising and falling" interconnectedness of all there is. As Buddhists have held for over a millennium, this alleged individual, solitary mind is an illusion from which we have profound difficulty freeing ourselves, though this liberation is the only path in awakening to our true nature. 'Mind' is rather an active engagement with the world, a process, not a static entity. Dumouchel and Damiano's analysis offers rich insight, for it pulls us out of our notion of an encapsulated, individualized, separate, private sense of bodiliness.

To a degree, Clark and Chalmers' thesis does as well. But Dumouchel and Damiano, in particular, open up the possibility of a social, interactive embodiment in that "our emotions and our empathic reactions are neither private productions not solitary undertakings." Moreover, "emotions are embodied in what may be called a 'social body.'"[41] In no way does this diminish the patient's private suffering. Instead, it situates it in the unique world of that patient's lived, embodied experience and, in turn, enables a patient's suffering to somehow be shared empathically. All this compels us to ask ourselves whether we are carting our Western philosophical prejudices to this discussion. If so, are we able to lay them aside and consider views such as the above that question the conventional assumptions of human exceptionalism as well as our bias regarding individual, separate selves? The human-robot interaction forces us to revisit our assumptions about who we are, how we think, what "mind" is, and how we relate to other living beings. Or will we hang on to that age-old sentimentality of holding on to our cognitive core, our minds, our "selves" as something absolutely distinct, separate, and irreducibly independent?

Throughout our lingering COVID-19 gauntlet, we have maintained connection with each other only through the redeeming power of our devices. They have been emancipating gifts from Prometheus. We have also grasped their limits. During those countless times when we needed to reach out to help relieve the anguish, pain, and suffering of loved ones, our devices could only go so far in enabling us to connect with others. Has misery awakened us to the perennial truth that nothing substitutes for a living flesh and blood touch and embrace? We yearn for that human-to-human, face-to-face connectedness. Again, this brings us back to that stubborn quest to discover the connections and caring we may possibly have from a caring robot. Like Talos, they can protect us under the menace of invasion, in our case, the threat of deadly, contagious pathogens. And like the mortal Talos, they have their flaws. Before we examine shortcomings, let us uncover more of their marvelous gifts.

NOTES

1. As I explain in the Introduction, each chapter begins with a retelling of a myth or legend. This is my rendition of the story of Talos as it is described in more detail in Adrienne Mayor, *Gods and Robots: Myths, Machines, and Ancient Dreams of Technology* (Princeton, NJ: Princeton University Press, 2018), 5–10.

2. Paul Ricoeur, *The Symbolism of Evil*, trans. Emerson Buchanan (New York: Harper & Row, 1967), 5.

3. Paul Ricoeur, *Time and Narrative*, Volume 3, trans. Kathleen Blamey and David Pellauer (Chicago: University of Chicago Press, 1988), 105.

4. Ricoeur, *Time and Narrative*, 105.

5. Ronald A. Heifetz and Donald L. Laurie, "The Work of Leadership," *Harvard Business Review* 5, no. 1 (January–February 1997): 124–34.

6. Paul Dumouchel and Luisa Damiano, *Living With Robots*, trans. Malcolm DeBevoise (Cambridge, MA: Harvard University Press, 2017), 102.

7. Nicholas A. Christakis, *Apollo's Arrow: The Profound and Enduring Impact of Coronavirus on the Way We Live* (New York: Little, Brown Spark, 2020), 167.

8. Michael C. Brannigan, "Does Seamus the Robot Care for Me?" *Times Union*, Feb. 27, 2011, https://www.timesunion.com/opinion/article/Does-Seamus-the-robot-care-for-me-1032481.php.

9. Nel Noddings, *Caring: A Feminine Approach to Ethics and Moral Education* (Berkeley: University of California Press, 1984), 24.

10. Adapted from Brannigan, "Does Seamus the Robot Care for Me?"

11. Christina Jewett, Shefali Luthra, and Melissa Bailey, "Federal Records Show Thousands of Desperate Pleas from Health Care Workers Seeking Better COVID Protective Gear," ABC News, June 30, 2020, https://abcnews.go.com/Health/federal-records-show-thousands-desperate-pleas-health-care/story?id=71530087.

12. Alex Chhith, "Dedicated Las Vegas Nurse with a 'Big Heart' Killed by COVID-19 at 39," *Las Vegas Review-Journal*, August 19, 2020, https://www.reviewjournal.com/local/local-las-vegas/dedicated-las-vegas-nurse-with-big-heart-killed-by-covid-19-at-39-2098596/.

13. Chhith, "Dedicated Las Vegas Nurse"; see also Christina Jewett, "'Lost on the Front Line': Tracks Health Workers Who Died of COVID-19," interview with Steve Innskeep, NPR Transcript, April 8, 2021, Audio, 06:00, https://www.npr.org/transcripts/985253407.

14. Jewett et al., "Federal Records Show Thousands of Desperate Pleas."

15. Jewett et al., "Federal Records Show Thousands of Desperate Pleas."

16. "U.S. Health Care from a Global Perspective, 2019: Higher Spending, Worse Outcomes?" *Commonwealth Fund Issue Brief*, Jan. 30, 2020, https://www.commonwealthfund.org/publications/issue-briefs/2020/jan/us-health-care-global-perspective-2019.

17. World Health Organization, "World Health Organization Coronavirus (COVID-19) Dashboard," accessed July 28, 2021, https://covid19.who.int/.

18. "COVID-19: Health care worker death toll rises to at least 17000 as organizations call for rapid vaccine rollout," Amnesty International, Mar. 5, 2021, https://www.amnesty.org/en/latest/news/2021/03/covid19-health-worker-death-toll-rises-to-at-least-17000-as-organizations-call-for-rapid-vaccine-rollout/.

19. "COVID-19: Health Care Worker Death Toll."

20. "COVID-19: Health Care Worker Death Toll."

21. Ellie Kincaid, "One Year into the Pandemic, More than 3,000 Healthcare Workers Have Died of COVID-19," *Medscape*, March 11, 2021, https://www.medscape.com/viewarticle/947304.

22. "Lost on the Frontline," *Guardian* and Kaiser Health News, April 8, 2021, https://www.theguardian.com/us-news/ng-interactive/2020/aug/11/lost-on-the-frontline-covid-19-coronavirus-us-healthcare-workers-deaths-database.

23. "Sir Luke Fildes the Doctor,'' Tate Gallery, accessed March 2021. https://www.tate.org.uk/art/artworks/fildes-the-doctor-n01522.

24. Cora Engelbrecht and Caroline Kim, "Zoom Shivas and Prayer Hotlines: Ultra-Orthodox Jewish Traditions Upended by Coronavirus," *New York Times*, April 16, 2020, https://www.nytimes.com/video/us/100000007061978/coronavirus-ultra-orthodox-jewish-traditions.html.

25. Engelbrecht and Kim, "Zoom Shivas and Prayer Hotlines."

26. Michael C. Brannigan, "Need for Face-to-Face Contact Transcends Viral Moment," *Times Union* May 28, 2020, https://www.timesunion.com/opinion/article/Need-for-face-to-face-contact-transcends-viral-15301656.php.

27. Renée C. Fox, *Experiment perilous: Physicians and Patients Facing the Unknown* (Glencoe, IL: Free Press, 1959).

28. Renée C. Fox, "The Evolution of Medical Uncertainty." *Milbank Memorial Fund Quarterly/Health and Society* 58, no. 1 (Winter 1980): 1.

29. Renée C. Fox and Judith P. Swazey, *The Courage to Fail: A Social View of Organ Transplants and Dialysis* (Chicago: University of Chicago Press, 1973), xiii-4.

30. Renée C. Fox, *In the Field: A Sociologist Journey* (New Brunswick, NJ: Transaction Publishers, 2011), 101.

31. Sherwin Nuland, *How We Die: Reflections of Life's Final Chapter* (New York: Alfred A. Knopf, 1994), 248–49.

32. Sherwin Nuland, *How We Die*, 248–49.

33. Bruno Latour, *Petites leçons de sociologie des sciences* (Paris: La Découverte, 2006).

34. Andy Clark and David Chalmers, "The Extended Mind." *Analysis* 58, no. 1 (January 1998): 7–19.

35. Clark and Chalmers, "The Extended Mind."

36. Andy Clark, *Natural-Born Cyborgs: Minds, Technologies, and the Future of Human Intelligence* (New York: Oxford University Press, 2003).

37. Dumouchel and Damiano, *Living With Robots*, 75–76.

38. Paul Humphreys, *Extending Ourselves: Computational Science, Empiricism, and Scientific Method* (New York: Oxford University Press, 2004).

39. Dumouchel and Damiano, *Living with Robots*, 85.

40. Dumouchel and Damiano, *Living with Robots*, 87.

41. Dumouchel and Damiano, *Living with Robots*, 141.

Chapter Two

Promise

From legendary accounts of his work in Athens, Crete, and Sicily, Daedalus was a craftsman par excellence, our original human inventor. Whether or not he was an actual historical person, he represents the archetype of imagination, discovery, and design, particularly novel technology to enhance human abilities and lifestyle. Samples of his tenacious engineering genius include construction of the hollow wooden cow designed to enable a bull to mate with Crete's Queen Pasiphae, resulting in the birth of a boy with a bull's head, the mythic Minotaur; the baffling labyrinth for King Minos of Crete; his exquisite honeycomb of gold with its perfect hexagonal geometry; mesmerizing waterworks and thermal baths; and his lifelike statues.[1] Daedalus is best known for designing wings for himself and his son Icarus to escape from King Minos' labyrinth and fly away, a tale we will later describe. He represents brilliant technological ingenuity. And we have inherited his marvelous capacity to invent new, sophisticated tools and to innovate in ways that no doubt boost our natural abilities, our tireless curiosity, eagerness to learn, and desire to reach beyond our limits.

Global pre-pandemic mental health was devastating, with the World Health Organization reporting over 250 million cases of depression. Since COVID-19 mushroomed, we have become further unhinged with higher rates of depression, burn-out, loneliness, and suicidal ideation. In the U.S., a recent Kaiser Foundation study revealed that, in 2019, 11 percent of Americans reported symptoms of anxiety and depression. Since the pandemic, that quickly escalated to 41 percent of American adults.[2] Many of them included our elders, particularly those who lived alone. In most cases their partners have died. Numerous others are alone in nursing homes. Before proceeding further, let me explain why I use the noun "elder." While the term seems dated and old-fashioned, in the past, "elder" referred to the respected and honored moral authority that comes with age and experience. In our youth-success-productivity oriented society, our treadmill use of "the elderly" means "old person" with its negative overtones. I propose resuscitating "elder" as a way of bestowing aging's inherent value and dignity, and as a way of restoring a cohesive philosophy of life stages which our culture so desperately lacks.

As for elders and all others living alone, social isolation jeopardizes physical and psychological health such as diminished immune systems, mounting blood pressure, cognitive decline, and depression. When the plague gained ground, The World Health Organization issued its "Mental health and psychosocial considerations during the COVID-19 Outbreak," a strong message to those who are isolated.

> Stay connected and maintain your social networks. Try as much as possible to keep your personal daily routines or create new routines if circumstances change. If health authorities have recommended limiting your physical social contact to contain the outbreak, you can stay connected via telephone, e-mail, social media or video conference.[3]

"Stay connected via telephone, e-mail, social media or video conference." The blessings of digital connectivity have become abundantly clear during the pandemic. This was the case well before the plague. A 2013 European study relating internet use among those over sixty-five found that regular use lessened the likelihood of social isolation, that, "personal social meetings and virtual contacts are complementary, rather than substituting for each other. Internet use may be a useful way of reducing social isolation."[4] No doubt, demography has ignited the urgency. With its population of over 126 million, seriously declining birth rates, and people living longer, Japan faces its "Silver Tsunami." There are simply not enough young people to care for their elders. With over 28 percent of its population over 65, Japan has the highest percentage of seniors worldwide. European countries face the same tidal wave of an aging population to be cared for with less people to care for them. Italy has the second highest percentage of seniors with 23 percent, followed by Portugal at 22.4 percent.[5] This is further compounded in view of pervasive chronic conditions that require ongoing care and monitoring.

What does it mean to care for these persons, especially elders and others with chronic illness? Caring for them is not simply about addressing the pathology of the underlying condition. It also means being sensitive to and understanding the web of relations in the person's social environment that contribute to a medical, social, interpersonal, and existential limbo, one that Arthur Kleinman terms "chronicity."[6] His description of "chronicity," written in 1988, powerfully resonates with us in the wake of our pandemic purgatory.

> It [chronicity] is the outcome of lives lived under constraining circumstances with particular relationships to other people. Chronicity is created in part out of negative expectations that come to be shared in face-to-face

interactions—*expectations that fetter our dreams and sting and choke our sense of self. Patients learn to act as chronic cases; family members and care givers learn to treat patients in keeping with this view* . . . The chronically ill often are like those trapped at a frontier, wandering confused in a poorly known border area, waiting desperately to return to their native land. Chronicity for many is the dangerous crossing of the borders, the interminable waiting to exit and reenter normal everyday life, the perpetual uncertainty of whether one can return at all. To pass through this world of limbo is to move through a 'nervous' system, a realm of menacing uncertainty.[7] (author emphasis)

Demography and chronicity is a deadly combination. Given the flood of those in desperate need of care and the shrinking numbers of those willing to offer care, caregiving for elders has unmistakably reached a watershed moment. With less people entering mental healthcare careers, robots can help fill the gap. Caring robots can also help caregivers, many of whom encounter high levels of burn-out and stress both from their work with elderly residents and with excessive institutional pressures. Through helping out with routine chores, robots can allow human caregivers to spend more time with those they should be caring for.

ROBOT WONDERS

There is no denying the vast benefits of robots. They help with tedious industrial work in our factories, household chores like the Roomba vacuum cleaner sweeping rugs, and yard duties like Robomow's Robotic Lawn Mower. Robots can take our blood pressure, play chess, assist in delicate surgery like the daVinci Surgical System, perform dangerous feats like exploring the surface of planets, and help clean up from disasters. Robots go where humans fear to tread. Since Japan's March 11, 2011 terrible earthquake, tsunami, and Fukushima Daiichi Nuclear Power Station meltdown, robots are still being used to clean up highly radiated debris and regularly assess contamination levels. They have saved lives detecting and dismantling explosive devices and in deep-sea recovery. Future developments may see robotic surgeons that can be used for a patient in one country via remote control from a physician in another country.

As Assistants

Companies developing caring robots place a premium on the safety, well-being, and satisfaction of the one cared-for. Moreover, they recognize the critical importance of a person's privacy and personal dignity. Carebots can reinforce these values by sustaining a patient's dignity, for example, when a person chooses to be cleaned by a carebot instead of feeling ashamed in front of another. Here is a sampling of the many robot assistants aimed to help vulnerable groups such as elders, disabled, and children with autism.

Georgia Institute of Technology has designed Cody, a robotic nurse. Cody can bath incapacitated elders and others who need help maintaining personal hygiene. What is especially important is that the patients whom Cody takes care of are not merely passive but remain active agents. Through voice command, patients themselves can control Cody's movements and pressure when, for instance, the robot washes parts of the body.[8] And we have robots specifically intended for family care. The U.S. GeckoSystems company is a pioneer in developing Mobile Service Robots (MSRs) for families who look after an elder or disabled family member. The company's CareBot™ is specifically designed to help family members and caregivers, especially with monitoring children with disabilities.[9] In Japan, Osaka University's roboticist Hiroshi Ishiguro has designed a tele-operated android, a robot assistant named Telenoid R1 to assist in elder care, particularly for residents in nursing homes. Through connecting remotely with the Telenoid, an operator transmits his or her voice and head movements to the Telenoid. We will discuss Ishiguro's creations in a later chapter, particularly his Geminoids. The Telenoid has a minimalist design, with a small child's body size, a doll-like, expressionless face, and nubs for hands and feet, with feet wrapped in soft fabric. Its minimalism suggests any gender and age, and its inexpressive face helps patients with cognitive decline project their feelings on to the robot. It also assists family members and care home staff in monitoring and communicating with the cared-for when they are away.[10] And let us not forget South Korea. The company Yujin Robot developed a multi-robot system with two bot platforms: iRobi and Cafero. With its childlike voice, the smaller iRobi acts as a receptionist to direct patients to healthcare services. It connects with the Cafero robot, and through its touchscreen, it enables user interaction with messages and pictures. Cafero reminds users about taking their medications and helps patients in measuring vital signs, blood pressure, blood oxygen, and pulse rate.[11] Having no need for rest, robots can monitor residents to remind them to take their medications on time, to look for behavioral warning signs like a change in the way someone walks, and to spot accidents and emergencies and alert the appropriate parties. Mitsubishi Heavy Industries developed its 3-foot robot Wakamaru as a companion for elders with its camera and integrated phone to monitor and alert authorities in an emergency. And in England, IBM Research U.K. has partnered with Cera Care to conduct studies on applying LiDAR sensor technology. Also used in autonomous cars, this detector apparatus keeps an 'eye' on seniors and the disabled to monitor their safety and alert authorities in emergencies. Are you concerned about grandma leaving pots and pans on a hot stove? According to Cera Care leaders Doctors Ansgar Lange and Ben Maruthappu, "While LiDAR promises to act as a powerful set of 'eyes and ears,' IBM Watson AI will provide the brains . . . and alert caregivers and medical personnel to possible deteriorations in a person's health (such as changes in gait) or emergency situations (such as a fall)."[12]

As Companions

Can carebots be companions? Companionship not in simply being-around, keeping an eye on me for medications, mishaps, etc. But companionship in a deeper sense of cultivating a relationship, a bonding in which I feel that my companion senses my state-of-being, my anxieties, apprehensions, someone with whom I can share my thoughts, someone who picks up on my signals. The possibility of a robot relating to me in this way is currently a formidable improbability. But, let us use our long-term imagination based in current directions in AI research and robotics. Will companionship in this sense be a viable option in the future? This was the vision over 20 years ago when the Cambridge, Massachusetts Company iRobot began designing interactive toys. Its animatronic doll My Real Baby came on the market in 2000. The doll not only babbles like a baby, but smiles and cries "Want baba!" to simulate hunger. It also says "uh oh" to call attention to a soiled diaper. M.I.T.'s Robert Brooks, chief technical officer of iRobot, asserts both the doll's fun aspect and its capacity to nurture a child's imagination, claiming "It's a toy which can enhance fantasy."[13]

Though this was the foresight in the U.S. two decades ago, robotics in Japan continues to lead the field in developing companion or "sociable robots." One of their earlier creations, a robot baby harp seal named Paro (priced at c. $6,000) is still used in homes for elders as companions, a "mental commitment robot" that can offer emotional support. Residents interact with it as if it was real. By sensing where a voice comes from, highly advanced technology enables real-time eye movements and vocalizations when Paro is being held and stroked. In her wonderfully insightful *Robo Sapiens Japanicus*, anthropologist Jennifer Robertson gives an in-depth account of robotics in Japan.[14] In measured fashion, she views robotics from a Japanese cultural lens. For instance, because its "father," Takanori Shibata, Paro's inventor, is Japanese-born, Paro was granted *koseki* (household status), equivalent to Japanese citizenship, in 2010.

Though this status is symbolic and not literal, Robertson gives a deft account of how this demonstrates the intertwining of robotics with Japan's traditional emphasis on family.[15] And there is the robot koala Wandakun, created by the Japanese company Matsushita. Like Paro, Wandakun responds to human touch with its eyes and its purring. Imagine someone who, feeling alone and alienated, after spending time with her pet baby seal or pet koala, feels more comfortable approaching others. "How are you today Marjorie? I'm feeling fine. I just had Paro with me this morning." Sony's AIBO robotic dog also responds to the human voice and responds to a number of commands. Priced at c. $3,000 and trendy in Japan when it first came out, the aibo, "pal" in Japanese, has the same kind of Organic Light Emitting Diodes (OLEDs) used for TV displays. With cameras in its nose and back and sensors on its body, it responds to touch. Its advanced artificial intelligence enables the companion dog to learn its owner's behavior and react accordingly. The aibo can take photos and adapt to smiles and other facial expressions. Intriguingly, a Buddhist temple in suburban Tokyo holds funeral services for robot dogs, considered by many Japanese as a beloved family companion.[16]

Seeking to outdo Sony's AIBO, South Korean company Dasarobot of Dasatech developed the bull terrier Genibo robot. The extremely popular Genibo is user-friendly, behaves as a lovable pet dog, wags its tail, and responds to simple voice commands. A company selling the robot (for $1,800 dollars) describes features including "autonomous behavior," "voice command recognition," "self reaction function," and "control manager" that can also be remote.[17]

Meet Kaspar. Robotic therapy for children with autism spectrum disorder has come a long way. The more recent KASPAR (Kinesics and Synchronisation in Personal Assistant Robots) stems from the work of Kerstin Dautenhahn and her research team at the U.K.'s University of Reading. Kaspar's neutral and simplified childlike face is deliberately designed to *not* respond in ways that appear reactive and judgmental. Its minimalist countenance enables a child to interact with it more freely. It responds to a child's interaction with no hint of anger or rejection. Its behavior is more simple and predictable than that of humans, and, absent the potential for shaming or embarrassment, KASPAR aids in nurturing a child's cognitive and social skills.[18]

With all this, robots can certainly offer a reassuring presence, being "present" enough for those with dementia to feel less anxiety. In Santa Clara, California, Tombot's new robotic therapy puppy, Jennie, inexpensively priced at under $500, is targeted for seniors with dementia.[19] With interactive sensors that detect touch and emits real puppy sounds as well as responds to voice commands, Jennie's mere physical presence can be comforting for the person being cared-for. This reassuring presence is sprinkled throughout Kazuo Ishiguro's *Klara and the Sun*, as Josie's artificial friend (AF) Klara takes great effort to be unobtrusive in the company of others. Klara is exceptionally perceptive, devoted to Josie. Klara is especially discreet when Josie is with her boyfriend Rick. Klara is simply there, in case Josie needs her, and Josie knows this. For Josie, this being present is in itself healing. When Josie became ill, the watchful and guarded housekeeper Melania allowed Rick to visit her. Klara describes her role.

> The first afternoon Rick was shown up to the bedroom, I started to leave in order to give privacy, but Melania Housekeeper stopped me on the landing, whispering: "No, artificial friend (AF)! You stay here. Make sure no hanky-panky."
>
> So it became normal for me to remain during Rick's visits, even though he sometimes looked towards me with go away eyes, and almost never addressed me, even to say hello or goodbye. Had Josie also made such go away signals, I wouldn't have remained, even after Melania Housekeeper's instruction. But Josie seemed happy about my presence—I even thought she took comfort from it—though she never included me in their conversations.
>
> I did my best to give privacy by remaining on the Button Couch and fixing my gaze over the fields. I couldn't help hearing what was being said behind me, and though I sometimes thought I shouldn't listen, I remembered it was my duty to learn as much about Josie as possible, and that by listening in this way, I might gather fresh observations otherwise unavailable to me.[20]

As Therapists

What about a robot acting as our therapist? Compared to human therapists and counselors, there are some pretty solid benefits. Having 24/7 access, there is no need for an appointment, and no reason to feel rushed. Considering the social stigma we still place on mental disorder, your therapist robot is without bias and judgement. You can bare your soul without shame or embarrassment. These therapists can be found through an iPhone app like the penguin chatbot Wysa. Wysa is an AI system that offers cognitive-behavioral therapy blended with professional human support. It tracks your mood and acts as your mindfulness coach. You can speak freely with Wysa anytime, and what you share is anonymous and secure.[21] And there is the start-up company focusing on designing digital therapeutics for mental health, Woebot Health. The company's Woebot, the newest in chatbot therapy, is a handy online tool with smartphone apps, a conversational artificial intelligence system developed with natural language processing, deep learning, neural networking, and predictive analytics.

Why share our deepest thoughts with a machine? Wouldn't we rather speak with a human? Not quite. In their 2020 survey of global workplace dynamics, Workplace Intelligence and Oracle reported that 68 percent of over 12,000 respondents preferred sharing their personal, intimate, emotional issues with a robot instead of with a human.[22] But can we really have a conversation with a device? And can our "therapist" genuinely offer that much-needed empathy? We will tackle these questions later on. For now, with AI's progress in linguistic algorithms like phrasing and diction, these and other chatbots offer enormous benefits in a field that, like caregiving, is seriously dwindling despite the clear and urgent need for more health professionals.[23]

The fallout from our pandemic is an ongoing tsunami of mental distress that has seized more people worldwide. Sadly, with our shrinking number of mental health professionals, we are poorly equipped to handle this crisis. But when the human face is not there to interact with us, we can turn to our devices. Even if this is not quite like human-to-human interaction, if we feel better sharing with Wysa and Woebot, is that not better than nothing? Or is it? Is it worse than having no human therapist? Aside from the ever-raging moral concerns of privacy, the ever-real threat of hackers, and the insidious menaces presented by universal online sharing, echoing the "Sharing is Caring" company mantra in Dave Eggers foreboding *The Circle*, does our relation to our machines slice away our own humanness? Are the devices to which we have become addicted a deceptive balm of comfort to help us with our addiction?

Contagion and Confinement

A term that has painfully come of age during our pandemic is not new. It surfaced during this century's earlier bouts of contagion, well before the Western African Ebola virus disease (EVD) epidemic from 2013–2016, the Middle East respiratory syndrome coronavirus (MERS) since 2012, and the 2002–2004 SARS (severe acute respiratory syndrome) outbreak. It reappears whenever civilizations have faced the scourge of plague and infectious epidemics. Quarantine. "Quarantine" stems from the Italian *quaranta*, meaning "forty." In the wake of the horrible 14th century Black Death, the bubonic plague that decimated one-third of Europe, facilities were built on islands outside of Venice so that incoming ships could sequester for forty days. The numerological significance of 40, representing trial and hardship, finds ample Biblical expression. In the Old Testament the Great Flood in Genesis lasted 40 days and nights (Genesis 7:12); Moses spent 40 days and nights on Mount Sinai before receiving the Ten Commandments (Exodus 24:18); the Israelites wandered in the wilderness for 40 years (Deuteronomy 8:2–5); the maximum number of lashes specified by Jewish Law that a man could receive for a crime is forty (Deuteronomy 25:3). In the New Testament Jesus was tempted in the desert for 40 days and nights (Matthew 4:2), and the 40-day period of Lent commemorates these 40 days; between Jesus' resurrection and ascension there were 40 days (Acts 1:3). Nowadays, though it does not last 40 days, quarantine is still a strict period of isolation and testing for at least two weeks. Here is where carebots can be incredibly useful. In confined sites during periods of contagion—ships, prisons, homeless sites, meatpacking plants and other tight work spaces, healthcare settings, nursing homes, and other close quarters—carebots, impervious to germs and viruses, could monitor individuals, remind them of isolation measures, and alert authorities if necessary.

Ships

Carebots would be invaluable when infections occur in confined and crowded areas, rife for super-spreading like cruise ships, sports arenas, fitness centers, music clubs, nursing homes, and metropolitan hospitals. Throughout the pandemic, major super-spreader environments have been prisons, nursing homes, close-quartered businesses like meatpacking plants, and settings like ships and cruises. As we know, ships were early hot zones, like the nuclear aircraft carrier USS *Theodore Roosevelt* with its crew of over of 4,700 on its way toward the western Pacific from its San Diego base. The COVID-19 outbreak, first discovered in March 2020, eventually infected over 1,200 sailors and killed one. When Captain Brett Crozier requested evacuating the ship due to the near impossibility of maintaining physical distance in such close quarters, he met with resistance from his superiors. His plan to clear the ship was somehow published in the *San Francisco Chronicle* after which he was summarily fired from his position by acting Secretary of Navy Thomas Modfly, who later resigned following public exposure and pressure. By that time most of the crew were ordered ashore, and Crozier eventually tested positive. The crew was mostly young and in good health. Many who tested positive never showed symptoms. The incident was a defining moment. It underscored the likelihood for both symptomatic and asymptomatic transmission of the virus, particularly in confined spaces and, because face coverings, hygiene, and distancing in themselves are not enough in such congregate settings, the critical need for ongoing testing.[24]

When the cruise ship Grand Princess embarked from San Francisco to Mexico and returned to San Francisco in late February 2020, most of the crew and passengers stayed on board as the ship then headed to Hawaii with over 2,300 new passengers. Within weeks in route, one passenger was found to have the novel coronavirus. The ship returned to port, making landfall March 8. All passengers and crew were then quarantined at military bases. seventy-eight were tested positive.

Those on board the Grand Princess and the USS *Theodore Roosevelt* were able to get ashore, off the ships. Not so with the Diamond Princess. On Feb. 5, 2020, after disembarking a few passengers who tested positive for COVID-19, the Diamond Princess, with over 3700 passengers and crew, remained quarantined in Yokohama Port, not allowed to disembark. Of the over 700 who contracted the virus, twelve died. This was the leading outbreak outside of China at that time. Among crew, most of those infected were food service workers. In a study to estimate the reproductive number (R0) of the virus during the early phases of the transmission on the ship, R0 "defined as the expected number of secondary cases that one primary case will generate in a susceptible population," the authors reported an estimated R0 of 2.28, heightening the need for immediate safeguards, monitoring, and testing at the very start.[25] In these confined settings, carebots could disinfect decks and other areas, bring food to the passengers, monitor the ship maintaining a sort of border control, and take vital signs and report results to health professionals on land.

Prisons

Prisons were also super-spreader settings. The U.S. accounts for just over 4 percent of the world's population. Yet it has more people in jails and prisons per capita than anywhere else on the planet, constituting nearly 25 percent of all those incarcerated.[26] Prisons are breeding grounds for infection. Their confinement forces inmates to work in taxingly crowded conditions. Though more protected in their cells, their daily routines—laundry, machine shop, workplace, etc.—often impose a suffocating closeness that makes physical distancing impractical. Prisons' rate of infection was explosive, second to nursing homes, with over 620,000 reported COVID cases. In a recent *New England Journal of Medicine* commentary arguing for increased measures of decarceration as a public health measure during the U.S. vaccine rollout, the authors state "Because there is constant movement in and out of jails and prisons . . . these facilities operate as epidemiologic pumps." Moreover, the authors not only anticipate a relatively high rate of vaccine hesitancy, but assert that, on account of the nature of the prison system and environment, vaccination in itself will not guarantee safety.

> In this setting, even a vaccine with 90 percent efficacy will leave many people at ongoing risk for Covid-19, given the extraordinarily high rate of transmission in jails and prisons attributable to rampant overcrowding, inadequate testing and health care, high-volume daily inflow and outflow of staff and detainees, lack of personal protective equipment, and normalized systematic neglect of the welfare of incarcerated people.[27]

Homeless

In contrast to prisons and ships, the homeless are not confined to any space. Their prisons are on the streets, under the bridges, in parks, and in alleyways. There are over 500,000 homeless persons in the U.S. They lack the safe harbor of a place where others can be there for them, the shelter that inmates have, and the caring environment of a nursing home. My friend Jim O'Connell is a physician who spearheads the pioneering work and mission of Boston Health Care for the Homeless Program. Its teams offer round-the-clock health services at numerous sites, shelters, soup kitchens, day centers, corrections facilities, and detoxification units, reaching out directly to homeless on the streets throughout the Boston area. It offers an innovative medical respite program to offer acute, recuperative, palliative, and end-of-life care. "Homeless" covers a wide swath of those marginalized in our communities. Committed to the consecrated challenge of healing, and who himself embodies empathy and compassion, Jim describes a group he calls "rough sleepers."

> Rough sleepers are an eclectic group of resolute individuals who embrace a modern brand of rugged American individualism and who eschew the rules and crowds of the shelters . . . Despite their ubiquitous presence on the urban American landscape, these impoverished individuals' tragic lives remain hidden and obscure . . . Despite an average age of only forty-five when our subjects first began this study, a third of these individual were dead within five years. The leading causes were cancer, heart disease, and liver disease . . . In a scathing rebuke of my own profession, Medicaid reported that these 119 individuals had an aggregate 18,383 emergency room visits in the five years between 1999 and 2003. We are only beginning to understand the ethical and financial costs of our society's neglect of those who live chronically on our streets without access to safe and affordable housing.[28]

Surge Capacity

Though not a super-spreader venue, hospital intensive care units (ICUs) with faulty ventilation and nebulizers have enabled the spread of viruses from ICU patients' secretions, adversely affecting frontline healthcare workers. As a general rule of thumb, hospitals are not safe places because of the potential for infection. This spread via aerosolization of viruses was clearly evident as well in meatpacking plants, nursing homes, and prisons. Here, having carebots, germ-proof and virus-proof, would be invaluable and save lives. From the start, the pandemic has raised crucial concerns about healthcare systems' capacity worldwide. Surge capacity has to do with situations when some sudden or unfolding crisis incurs present and potential large-scale injury that brings about a drastic need for medical needs, supplies, resources, personnel, and support. This surge in demand overwhelms existing medical capabilities in emergency units and intensive-care units, ICUs.[29] Surge capacity is a precarious stew involving the following ingredients. 1) What is our hospital bed capacity? The U.S. rates low per capita compared to other countries. Its

2.9 beds per thousand people is disconcerting compared to S. Korea's 11.5 beds per thousand.[30] 2) What about ICU beds? The U.S. has over 100,000 ICU beds. That may seem high. But look at the numbers. We have suffered over 600,000 fatalities from COVID-19, with many victims in dire need of ICU treatment. Over 30 million Americans were infected with COVID. If only 1 percent of them needed ICU beds, that would be 300,000 beds, well over what we have.[31] 3) Do we have enough healthcare workers to handle the surge, including doctors, nurses, staff, cleaners, etc. 4) What about our available supply of personal protective equipment including masks and respirators? 5) What do we have in terms of medical equipment such as ventilators, etc.? 6) Do we have enough units to deal hygienically with corpses—coffins, refrigeration, mortuary capacity, etc.? Carebots cannot fill the need for many of these. But, by working in direct contact and close quarters with infected patients, they can help ease the appalling burden healthcare workers face, and to help alleviate fears of transmission and use of scarce medical resources.

ARTIFICIAL INTELLIGENCE PAVES THE WAY

In 2017, Xiaoyi, "little doctor," became the world's first robot to pass the medical licensing exam in China, and with high grades. This was its second attempt. But Xiaoyi did its homework digesting all sorts of information from medical textbooks and countless medical records and articles. The exam does not just require rote memorization, but medical reasoning, processing patient data, and forming decisions. The Chinese start-up company iFlyTek, in collaboration with Tsinghua University, developed Xiaoyi to be a doctor's assistant to collect and assess patient data. The robot's team consisted not only of engineers but medical professionals who offered their experiential input for the robot's AI algorithms. With all-out research on AI-driven robots and AI technologies, China may become the world leader in AI development within decades. iFlyTek's chairman, Liu Qingfeng, tells us, "Rather than replacing doctors, AI is able to help doctors better serve patients . . . By studying the medical cases and diagnosis skills of top doctors in top hospitals in megacities in China, our doctor AI can serve as an assistant to help doctors in remote areas in the country."[32] This may all sound strange to us unless we are already familiar with Baidu, Alibaba, and Tencent, China's versions of Google, Amazon, and Facebook respectively. Nonetheless, iFlytek is walking the talk and working full force in AI applications like speech and facial recognition for medicine for a growing number of Chinese hospitals.

AI's Quiet Success

Artificial intelligence platforms paved the way to robots for quite some time. The path did not just pop up in 2011 when IBM's Watson trounced human champions Ken Jennings and Brad Rutter in Jeopardy. It was paved long before in an all-out, persistent effort to produce a thinking machine that would not only match the human brain but surpass it. As a result, computer power has far outpaced human skills, for example in sports and chess. As Erik Brynjolfsson and Andrew McAfee reveal in their virtuoso *The Second Machine Age*, its appetite continues to be unquenchable with zetabytes of data churning out mega-mountains of information through byzantine algorithms. Its steady exponential explosion makes AI progress a combined sprint and marathon without a finish line.[33] AI's infiltration in our lives has been quiet and relentless, and now are we realizing more of its ubiquitous presence and power. While computer scientist John McCarthy named the infant "artificial intelligence" in the 1950s, its gestation reaches further back. AI has now come to be an umbrella term covering various subtypes, like a network based on Bayesian theorem that, when applied to medicine, deduces certain probable diagnoses, indicating the likelihood of each one after sifting through all the evidence and symptoms.[34] Especially in medicine, AI resembles an archaeological dig, excavating data, scouring through the existing medical literature which no human can keep up with, and arriving at an accurate diagnosis after filtering through the test data and vital medical information comprising output from datasets in tests, images, sensors, patient history, and genome sequencing. Here are examples of some of the riches from this archaeological dig.

With a relatively high rate of missed diagnoses in the U.S. by dermatologists, AI can be extremely valuable in accurately assessing skin conditions. AI algorithms using deep neural networking (DNN, computational networks of interconnected elements) in detecting skin cancer can clearly outperform human dermatologists.[35] For ophthalmologists, retinal images convey much about the state of the body. AI neural network can improve the accuracy of eye exams through optical coherence tomography (OCT), an ultrasound approach to an optical biopsy, using light instead of sound. Providing cross-sectional tissue images in real time, it is safer than the more invasive excisional biopsy. It is also invaluable in detecting signs for diabetic neuropathy and age-related macular degeneration (AMD).[36]

Medicine's digitization via AI has spurred what Eric Topol calls "deep medicine." His "deep medicine" comprises three components: deep phenotyping, deep learning, and deep empathy.[37] The first two are matters of technical aptitude. Deep phenotyping, what Topol describes as "digitizing the medical essence of a human being," involves digging into an individual's biology and history, medical and familial. One single person's life-data is massive considering multi-layers of DNA, RNA, proteins, etc. Deep learning is an amalgam of sophisticated pattern recognition and machine learning that promises untold benefits in healthcare settings. Remotely, it monitors individuals in their homes, thus reducing hospital visits. It delivers super proficiency in pattern recognition, one of the fundamental cornerstones of learning. As pointed to above, deep learning in medicine surpasses the technical capabilities of experts like radiologists, cardiologists, dermatologists, and ophthalmologists who assess images and data from medical tests. His third component is the most crucial—deep empathy and connection between providers and their patients. More to the heart of this book and one which we will later address, it concerns the degree to which our interface with machines cultivate genuine connectedness.

AI Wonders

Will robots replace surgeons? Not in the near future. However, scholars at Oxford and Yale universities surveyed what AI experts believe about future AI progress and probable timelines for when machines might replace or come close to supplanting humans in selected occupations. According to their report, robots could replace surgeons by mid-century.[38] What about other occupations? "Researchers predict AI will outperform humans in many activities in the next ten years, such as translating languages (by 2024), writing high-school essays (by 2026), driving a truck (by 2027), working in retail (by 2031), writing a bestselling book (by 2049), and working as a surgeon (by 2053)."[39]

When I was diagnosed with upper tract urothelial carcinoma, assigned a rather grim stage three with a high-grade tumor mass in my kidney lining, I underwent laparoscopic surgery to remove my left kidney and ureter. I was personally introduced to the da Vinci method. Dr. Ted Chang, known for his mastery of the da Vinci tool, performed the procedure. Both Dr. Chang and my oncologist Dr. David Shaffer were not only gifted experts, but genuine caregivers who represent the best of the best in professional and morally competent care. I was blessed. There are over 8 million surgical procedures performed annually in the U.S. Although not used in all types of surgeries, Intuitive Surgical Company's da Vinci Surgical System had been pioneering robotic surgery for nearly two decades. The da Vinci System is now in good company. More enterprises are developing AI-assisted robotic surgery to a point where, though still a far cry from ousting human surgeons, robotic surgical assistants now include robotic "surgeons" like the U.K.'s Cambridge Medical Robotics' "Versius," a robot with humanlike arms, Auris Health's endoscopic robot, nanotechnological development of robotic-assisted microsurgery for the human eye, and robots with advanced haptic touch sensors. Touch is our most human way to connect, feel, and learn, so developing touch sensors in a robot has profound implications.[40] AI surgery assistance promises to become more of a team effort with other AI systems. In 2015, Google and Johnson & Johnson collaborated in developing Verb Surgical, enabling distant robotic domains to connect with each other in real time during an actual surgery. This is like playing tennis and having various data about your opponent—weak spots, mental state, heart rate, tired strokes, shaky court positions—filtered to your wrist band and whispered to you as a bolt of advice for your next serve. As one study points out, a Verb Surgical robot "democratizes" surgery.[41]

In emergency medicine, time is uncompromising. After a stroke, for every minute a blood clot in the brain, or vessel occlusion, hinders blood flow, a person loses around 2 million brain cells. Early diagnosis of the possibility and degree of a stroke is therefore crucial. In 2018, the FDA approved the Lucid Robotic System, developed by Neural Analytics Inc. of Los Angeles. When paramedics arrive at a scene, this system enables them to quickly diagnose the severity of a stroke to better determine potential treatment. Paramedics place the robotic system on the patient's head. With its transcranial ultrasound and AI pattern recognition, the system sends ultrasound waves to the brain and transmits its findings to the hospital. Doctors can then meet the patient immediately upon entry. Head of neurology at Henry Ford Health System in Detroit, Stephan A. Mayer, claims that "This is potentially a breakthrough . . . The huge question in stroke care has been making a pre-hospital diagnosis of a large-vessel occlusion."[42]

AI voice platforms have clear advantages over writing. The oral tradition that long pre-dated the invention of writing and the later seismic revolutionary technology of printing is richly steeped in meaning. Both voice and writing remain subject to near infinite iteration and interpretation. And whether we engage with a screen, keyboard, cube, or cylinder, they are still objects. So can we have a real connection with an object? Nonetheless, voice platforms with their deep neural network technology are efficient, fast, and clean, even for the deaf. According to DNN expert Lars Bramslaw and audiologist Douglas Beck,

> The idea of a DNN within a computer chip is admittedly difficult to grasp. However, computer-based, pragmatic, and integrated DNNs are all around us. They have been used, and are particularly well-suited to, make sense of "big data." DNNs are currently being applied in many ways behind the scenes to allow computers to perform tasks which were once exclusively human tasks, such as:

- Automatic speech recognition
- Facial recognition
- Language translation
- Image enhancement
- Automatic handwriting identification
- Streamed music auto-select functions
- Drones delivering packages in crowded neighborhoods, and
- Self-driving cars.[43]

Just think of the 600,000 children and 3 million seniors in the U.S. who are visually impaired and blind, and the 780 million adults worldwide who are illiterate. These voice platforms can be marvelously beneficial. They can act as home aides, dictating messages, informing about TV shows, etc.[44]

With over 2 million biomedical articles published yearly, AI offers a technically feasible way to sift through all this and apply relevant research for patients for their own use on mobile apps. We are all potential patients, so having mobile apps with which we can check troubling symptoms is a boon. Boston's Buoy Health Inc., founded in 2014, developed its Symptom Checker that helps people self-diagnose their symptoms as soon as they experience them. Online self-diagnosis can be a tortuous tangle of confusing messages. Recognizing the uniqueness of each individual person, BuoyHealth is a digital tool, similar to a doctor's consult, that goes beyond the traditional decision tree analysis to more accurately help someone get a better sense of their condition and proper treatment.[45] Another promising venture is for doctors throughout the world to use their mobile apps for consults and suggestions from experts. The Human Diagnosis Project's Human Dx app aims to effectively apply machine learning algorithms, natural language processing, and physician crowdsourcing from over 10,000 physicians in 80 countries. Physicians can test their differential diagnoses by consulting with a specialist or group of medical peers. After input, the system then offers its final ranking of likely diagnoses. Human Dx ensures a way to address widespread lack of equitable access to health expertise, allowing patients to benefit from an international circle of specialists.[46]

AliveCor, headquartered in Mountain View, Calif., is a pioneer in consumer electrocardiogram technology (ECG). The company starred in the FDA's landmark November 30, 2017 approval of its AI algorithm that would enable consumers to self-monitor for a medical diagnosis. After trial and error, AliveCor developed its Kardia band which uses its AI algorithm to monitor heart rate and detect early signs for a possible atrial fibrillation (AFib) that could signal a stroke. The Kardia band detects atrial fibrillation and normal sinus rhythm. Not to be outdone, in the following September Apple announced its own FDA approved algorithm to detect atrial fibrillation as part of its Apple Watch series 4. But then in April 2019, AliveCor announced FDA clearance for two additional indications: to detect and show ECG results for bradycardia (slow heart beat, 40–50 beats/minute) and tachycardia (fast heart beat, 100–140 beats/minute). KardiaMobile, when paired with the Kardia app, provides instant analysis for detecting atrial fibrillation, bradycardia, tachycardia, and normal rhythm in an ECG. It is an invaluable tool for self-monitoring, patient empowerment, and informing clinicians in time regarding early detection of atrial fibrillation.[47]

Care.coach

Welcome to Care.coach, a fabulous, frontrunner service in digital caregiving that makes solid sense, and a good example of the kind of human-machine balance we will discuss in our last chapter. MIT mechanical engineering graduate Victor Wang, together with fellow MIT graduate in computer science Shuo Deng, co-founded this hybrid human-digital program in 2012 to help seniors, particularly those facing cognitive and memory challenges. A year earlier, Wang's grandmother was diagnosed with Lewy body dementia. Lewy body dementia results in a progressive decline in muscle and mental abilities. Similar to Alzheimer's Disease, symptoms include slowed and impaired muscle movement, autonomic nervous system irregularities, visual hallucinations, impaired regulation of body functions, cognitive, sleep, and attention disorders, and depression. His grandmother's condition sparked in him the idea of offering comfort to her and others remotely through a digital screen conduit. She and all others in need of caregiving far exceed available human caregivers. Think of 79 to 1. Writes Lauren Smiley for *Wired*, "between 2010 and 2030, the population of those older than 80 is projected to rise 79 percent but the number of family caregivers available is expected to increase just 1 percent."[48] Care.coach is specifically devoted to helping seniors. Its conversational platform engages seniors and assists users in enabling their self-management of chronic conditions, and provides compassionate support. Its cost-effectiveness, accessibility, and user-friendly interface makes it appealing for those confined to their home settings. In 2018, Care.coach was named one of four entrepreneurial winners of the In Good Company Optimal Aging Challenge, sponsored by the MIT AgeLab, which states:

> Researchers at universities and clinicians in diverse care settings have validated Care.coach's innovative approach in caregiving and its ability to reduce loneliness, improve perceived social support, and drive outcomes—including reducing the need for nursing visits to the home, preventing falls, and mitigating delirium among hospitalized older adults.[49]

Care.coach provides an app with a voice-assistant puppy avatar that speaks with and monitors users. The puppy is the digital face of the company's trained human care team like 35-year-old Rodrigo Rochin, in Monterrey, Mexico. Hence, humans and machines work together. Rodrigo is the eyes and voice behind the service's avatar, one of the company's human coaches who act behind the scenes, plying the app's AI audio and visual stream while interacting with the user. The user may or may not know he is there. Instead, the user interacts with the puppy on the screen while Rodrigo remains invisible. He is the eyes and voice of the avatar, meticulously taking notes on his clients with whom he builds a close relationship. Moreover, his work is collaborative. He keeps a log that is shared with the user's social workers and caregivers as well as with adult children of the user, all in an effort to help coordinate care. At the same time, by monitoring the activity of the human caregiver, he can notify the children of any questionable incidents. Care.coach's conversational platform reminds users of their meals, regular hydration, and medicine. It clearly helps human caregivers and in-home aides in their daily grind of caregiving, no easy task. The monthly cost of this continuous, accessible digital coach, around $200, is trifling compared to the monthly costs of regular nursing care, in-home and in residences. One of Rodrigo's clients, Jim, in his early 90s, named his puppy avatar Pony. Unbeknownst to Jim, Rodrigo acts the part of Pony.

> Sometimes Pony would hold up a photo of Jim's daughters or his inventions between his paws, prompting him to talk about his past. The dog complimented Jim's red sweater and cheered him on when he struggled to buckle his watch in the morning. He reciprocated by petting the screen with his index finger, sending hearts floating up from the dog's head. "I love you, Jim!" Pony told him a month after they first met—something CareCoach operators often tell the people they are monitoring. Jim turned to Arlyn [Jim's daughter] and gloated, "She does! She thinks I'm real good!"[50]

Is There an Algorithm for Caring?

"'ALGORITHM' IS A WORD whose time has come," writes history of science scholar Massimo Mazzotti, who goes on to claim that "Algorithms are changing the worlds we inhabit—and they're changing us."[51] In their simplest form, algorithms are sets of instructions or rules. They are often more intricate, detailed schema of crucial processes of how we do things. They are used in virtually all fields, but especially undergird AI and its super computations. Algorithms form the DNA of AI. But it is more than a simple formula or set of inner instructions for computers.

> We rarely use the word "algorithm" to refer solely to a set of instructions. Rather, the word now usually signifies a program running on a physical machine—as

well as *its effects on other systems*. Algorithms have thus become agents, which is partly why they give rise to so many suggestive metaphors. Algorithms now *do* things. They determine important aspects of our social reality. They generate new forms of subjectivity and new social relationships. They are how a billion-plus people get where they're going. They free us from sorting through multitudes of irrelevant results. They drive cars. They manufacture goods. They decide whether a client is creditworthy. They buy and sell stocks, thus shaping all-powerful financial markets. They can even be creative.[52]

Because of their pervasiveness and power, Massimo thinks of algorithms as "black-boxed."

> To black-box a technology is to turn it into a taken-for-granted component of our life—in other words, to make it seem obvious and unproblematic. The technology is thus shielded from the scrutiny of users and analysts, who cease seeing it as contingent and modifiable, accepting it instead as a natural part of the world.[53]

Our faith in the ubiquitous power of algorithms ultimately relies on our faith in the data that is fed to them. And human-guided algorithms, grounded on human input, is distinct from machine-guided algorithms, with input derived by machines. Take the matter of predictability. When his wife was diagnosed with breast cancer, multibillionaire Eric Lefkovsky realized how a dire lack of sufficient data hindered accurate cancer detection. Co-founder of Groupon, he formed Tempus Labs, a high-efficiency company using AI to develop more precise methods of machine learning, imaging analytics, natural language processing, and "deep phenotyping" to identify early signs of cancer. The company collaborates with over forty National Cancer Institute centers in the U.S.[54] As described earlier, medicine is a domain of uncertainty. Yet, with AI deep neural networks, uncertainty in predicting medical outcomes with specificity is thinning. AI algorithms can now predict a patient's death with more than 70 percent accuracy, often out-predicting humans. This will no doubt impact palliative care, the length of hospital stays, and insurance.[55] However, when it comes to end-of-life matters, the quantified clinical terrain is vastly distinct from the human landscape. Here, patients, families, spouses, and partners make real human choices, such as living out one's days at home, in a hospital, or hospice setting. There is no algorithm for these choices. And while our human choices will still be influenced by clinical metrics, remember the Riddle, the immense complexity in medical diagnosis. We humans can suffer from any one or more of 10,000 possible diseases. Reaching the correct diagnosis is no walk in the park. Furthermore, as Amos Tversky and Daniel Kahneman pointed out in their landmark study on unconscious cognitive biases, circumstances of uncertainty are also feeding grounds for cognitive bias.[56]

At heart is human fallibility. We touched upon this in our Introduction. For instance, our eyes are our most volatile and vulnerable organ. Yet, we can easily miss what is in front of us, especially when we are focused on looking for something else. Hence, the gorilla missed by most subjects who were instructed to count the number of ball passes among players.[57] Our eyes are absolutely crucial in specialties like radiology. The radiologist is the person patients usually never meet, yet who profoundly influences their lives by what he or she sees on their CT, MRI, PET, X-ray images, etc. When IBM acquired the medical imaging firm Merge Healthcare in 2015, it acquired access to over 30 billion images.[58] It will not be long before AI algorithms step in with an accuracy, efficiency, and speed that will place the human specialist's job at risk. The potential to dig deeper and prevent unnecessary treatments is vast and cannot be overstated. These AI wonders are, without doubt, invaluable and lifesaving. At the same time, they compel us to ask whether a patient, a person with moral agency, is ultimately measurable. Is the patient's medical persona her essence, her personhood? Eric Topol poses a similar question in the context of electronic health records, EHRs.

> We know there's much more data and information about a given person that is found in the EHR. There are medial encounters from other health systems and providers. There are antecedent illnesses and problems when the individual was younger or living in another place. There are data from sensors, like blood pressure, heart rhythm, or glucose, that are not entered in the chart. There are genomic data that millions of people have obtained that are not integrated into the record. And there is the social media content from networks like Facebook that goes ignored, too. Even if clinicians could work well with a patient's EHR, it still provides a very narrow, incomplete view.[59]

As we will see in the next chapter, the metamorphosis of the real patient to the so-called iPatient, charted and measured according to EHR template and algorithms, illustrates the unhealthy truncation in an algorithmic determinism of human persons.

This spurs us to inquire further—What then is the principal aim and purpose of medicine? Of caring? How do the two relate? And what about nurses, those on the front lines engaged in trench warfare with an invisible enemy throughout our pandemic committed to their missions to care. Will robots replace nurses? Though the jury is still out on this, the scales weigh heavily in favor of human nurses. Robots will no doubt take over quite a few caregiving tasks—monitoring patients, particularly in the ICU, taking vital signs, heart rate, and blood pressure, etc. But these are caregiving *tasks*. *Doing* these tasks does not mirror a caregiver's disposition, attitude, and degree of empathy. Ideally they match up, but these essentials are not quite like human-to-human caring. Only through asking ourselves about the essential purpose in medicine and healthcare can we reasonably establish what patients and persons being cared-for genuinely seek and need. How we respond shapes what we *expect* in the dynamic engagement between physician and patient, caregiver and cared-for, whether we think of it as solely contractual, commercially fixed, a matter of performance, or as something more, involving a moral glue that tightens the relational bond.

This then demands revisiting the purpose of medicine, digging into its fundamental *telos*. Arthur Kleinman offers us a look at what this reconceptualizing of medical care incurs, one that conveys the weighty challenge facing caregivers. Genuine care involves,

> (1) empathic witnessing of the existential experience of suffering and (2) practical coping with the major psychosocial crises that constitute the menacing chronicity of the experience. The work of the practitioner includes the sensitive solicitation of the patient's and the family's stories of the illness, the assembling of a mini-ethnography of the changing contexts of chronicity, informed negotiation with alternative lay perspectives on care, and what amounts to a brief medical psychotherapy for the multiple, ongoing threats and losses that make chronic illness so profoundly disruptive.[60]

Genuine care is more than performance. Taking *care of* another is distinct from *caring for and about* the other. Caring demands a moral commitment. As such, caring is and always should be the pulse of healthcare. Will carebots be up to the task? Or, more precisely, will they be designed to meet the challenge?

NOTES

1. This is again my retelling of the myth of Daedalus. The source is Adrienne Mayor, *Gods and Robots: Myths, Machines, and Ancient Dreams of Technology* (Princeton, NJ: Princeton University Press, 2018), 70–72, 85–90.

2. Nirmita Panchal et al., "The Implications of COVID-19 for Mental Health and Substance Use," Kaiser Family Foundation Study, February 10, 2021, accessed April 2021, https://www.kff.org/coronavirus-covid-19/issue-brief/the-implications-of-covid-19-for-mental-health-and-substance-use/.

3. "Mental Health and Psychosocial Considerations during the COVID-19 Outbreak," World Health Organization, March 18, 2020, 5, accessed 2 April 2020, https://www.who.int/docs/default-source/coronaviruse/mental-health-considerations.pdf?sfvrsn=6d3578af_2.

4. Orsolya Lelkes, "Happier and Less Isolated: Internet Use in Old Age," *Journal of Poverty and Social Justice* 21, no. 1 (February 2013): 33–46.

5. "Elderly citizens accounted for record 28.4 percent of Japan's population in 2018, data show," *The Japan Times*, Sept. 15, 2019, https://www.japantimes.co.jp/news/2019/09/15/national/elderly-citizens-accounted-record-28-4-japans-population-2018-data-show/#.Xjs3XKZYZPY.

6. Arthur Kleinman, *The Illness Narratives: Suffering, Healing, and the Human Condition* (New York: Basic Books, 1988), 80–81.

7. Kleinman, *The Illness Narratives*, 80, 81.

8. "Robotic Cody learns to bathe," *Georgia Tech College of Engineering,* Nov. 11, 2010, https://coe.gatech.edu/news/2010/11/robotic-cody-learns-bathe.

9. Mountain Marketing, Inc., "Family and Health Care Near Term Markets," Mar. 11, 2013, accessed Feb. 2021, https://www.geckosystems.com/investors/GeckoSystems-Family_and_Health_Care_Markets.pdf.

10. Erico Guizzo, "Telenoid R1: Hiroshi Ishiguro's Newest and Strangest Android," *IEEE Spectrum*, Aug. 1, 2010, https://spectrum.ieee.org/automaton/robotics/humanoids/telenoid-r1-hiroshi-ishiguro-newest-and-strangest-android.

11. Min Ho Lee1, Ho Seok Ahn, and Bruce A. MacDonald, "A Case Study: Robot Manager for Multi-Robot Systems with Heterogeneous Component-Based Framework," Australian Robotics and Automation Association paper, https://www.araa.asn.au/acra/acra2015/papers/pap139.pdf.

12. Ansgar Lange and Ben Maruthappu, "Could Autonomous Car Technology and AI Transform Home Care for the Elderly? IBM Think Blog, May 23, 2019, https://www.ibm.com/blogs/think/2019/05/could-autonomous-car-technology-and-ai-transform-homecare-for-the-elderly.

13. Katie Hafner, "A Robot That Coos, Cries and Knows When It Needs a New Diaper,*"* *New York Times,* Nov. 16, 2002, https://www.nytimes.com/2000/11/16/technology/a-robot-that-coos-cries-and-knows-when-it-needs-a-new-diaper.html.

14. Jennifer Robertson, *Robo sapiens japanicus: Robotos, Gender, Family, and the Japanese Nation* (Oakland: University of California Press, 2018).

15. Robertson, *Robo sapiens japanicus*, 137–41.

16. Levi Sumagaysay, "Sony's Aibo Robotic Dog Can Sit, Fetch and Learn What Its Owner Likes," *The Mercury News,* Sept. 24, 2018, https://phys.org/news/2018-09-sony-aibo-robotic-dog-owner.html.

17. Solvelight Robotics, "Genibo SD Companion Robot Dog," accessed Jan. 2021, https://www.solvelight.com/product/dst-robot-genibo-robot-dog/.

18. Paul Dumouchel and Luisa Damiano, *Living with Robots,* trans. Malcolm DeBevoise (Cambridge, MA: Harvard University Press, 2017), 162.

19. Keith Shaw, "Tombot Robotic Service Dog Wins 2019 Pitchfire, Hearts of Audience," *Robotics Business Review*, Oct. 3, 2019, https://www.roboticsbusinessreview.com/events/tombot-robotic-service-dog-wins-2019-pitchfire-hearts-of-audience.

20. Kazuo Ishiguro, *Klara and the Sun* (New York: Alfred A. Knopf, 2021), 117–18.

21. Wysa, accessed March 2021, https://www.wysa.io/.

22. "Global Study: 82 percent of People Believe Robots Can Support Their Mental Health Better Than Humans," Oracle News Connect, Oct. 7, 2020, https://www.oracle.com/news/announcement/ai-at-work-100720.html.

23. Michael C. Brannigan, "On Robots, Depression, and the Lure of the Not-Quite-Real," *Times Union*, April 1, 2021.

24. Mary Van Beusekom, "COVID-19 Spread Freely Aboard USS Theodore Roosevelt, Report Shows," CIDRAP News, University of Minnesota, Center for Infectious Disease Research and Policy, Oct 01, 2020, https://www.cidrap.umn.edu/news-perspective/2020/10/covid-19-spread-freely-aboard-uss-theodore-roosevelt-report-shows.

25. Sheng Zhang et al., "Estimation of the Reproductive Number of Novel Coronavirus (COVID-19) and the Probable Outbreak Size on the Diamond Princess Cruise Ship: A Data-Driven Analysis," *International Journal of Infectious Diseases* 93 (April 2020):201–204. See the HBO documentary "The Last Cruise," debuted early April 2021.

26. Benjamin A. Barsky et al., "Vaccination Plus Decarceration—Stopping Covid-19 in Jails and Prisons," *The New England Journal of Medicine* 384 (April 29, e, 2021):1583–1585.

27. Barsky et al., "Vaccination Plus Decarceration."

28. James J. O'Connell, *Stories from the Shadows* (Boston, MA: BHCHP Press, 2015), 128–29.

29. Michael C. Brannigan, *Japan's March 2011 Disaster and Moral Grit: Our Inescapable In-between* (Lanham, MD: Lexington Books, 2015), xx.

30. Nicholas A. Christakis, *Apollo's Arrow: The Profound and Enduring Impact of Coronavirus on the Way We Live* (New York: Little, Brown Spark, 2020), 92.

31. Christakis, *Apollo's Arrow*, 91–92.

32. Kimberley Mok, "Robot Passes a Medical Licensing Exam for the First Time Ever," *The Newstack*, Dec. 7, 2017, https://thenewstack.io/robot-passes-medical-licensing-exam-first-time-ever/.

33. Erik Brynjolfsson and Andrew McAfee, *The Second Machine Age: Work, Progress, and Prosperity in a Time of Brilliant Technologies* (New York, NY: W.W. Norton Company, Inc., 2014).

34. Robert Wachter, *The Digital Doctor: Hope, Hype, and Harm at the Dawn of Medicine's Computer Age* (New York: McGraw-Hill Education, 2015), 99.

35. Andre Esteva et al., "Dermatologist-level classification of skin cancer with deep neural networks," *Nature* 542 (Feb. 2017): 115–118, https://doi.org/10.1038/nature21056.

36. James G. Fujimoto et al., "Optical Coherence Tomography: An Emerging Technology for Biomedical Imaging and Optical Biopsy," Neoplasia 2, no. 1–2 (Jan. 2000): 9–25, https://doi.org/10.1038/sj.neo.7900071. See also Eric Topol, *Deep Medicine: How Artificial Intelligence Can Make Healthcare Human Again* (New York: Basic Books, 2019), 147.

37. Eric Topol, *Deep Medicine: How Artificial Intelligence Can Make Healthcare Human Again* (New York: Basic Books, 2019), 15f.

38. Katja Grace et al., "When Will AI Exceed Human Performance? Evidence from AI Experts," arXiv, May 3, 2018, https://arxiv.org/pdf/1705.08807.pdf.

39. Grace et al., "When Will AI Exceed Human Performance?" 1.

40. Topol, *Deep Medicine*, 161.

41. Topol, *Deep Medicine*, 161.

42. Thomas M. Burton, "New Stroke Technology to Identify Worst Cases Gets FDA Approval," *The Wall Street Journal*, May 30, 2018, https://www.wsj.com/articles/new-stroke-technology-to-identify-worst-cases-gets-fda-approval-1527709670.

43. Lars Bramsløw and Douglas L. Beck, "Deep Neural Networks in Hearing Devices," *Hearing Review.Com*, Special Issue, Hearing Aids and Cognition, January 2021: 29, https://www.ilhearing.org/assets/Education/2021/Bramslow%20Beck%20-%20Deep%20Neural%20Networks%20in%20Hearing%20Devices.pdf.

44. Topol, *Deep Medicine*, 260.

45. Buoy Health, accessed May 2021, https://www.buoyhealth.com/.

46. MacArthur Foundation, "Human Diagnosis Project," accessed March 2021, https://www.macfound.org/press/semifinalist-profile/human-diagnosis-project.

47. AliveCor, "FDA Grants First-Ever Clearances to Detect Bradycardia and Tachycardia on a Personal ECG Device," *Cision PR Newswire*, Apr. 23, 2019, https://www.prnewswire.com/news-releases/fda-grants-first-ever-clearances-to-detect-bradycardia-and-tachycardia-on-a-personal-ecg-device-300835949.html.

48. Lauren Smiley, "What Happens When We Let Tech Care for Our Aging Parents," *Wired*, Dec. 19, 2017, https://www.wired.com/story/digital-puppy-seniors-nursing-homes/.

49. Adam Felts, "MIT AgeLab Hosts Governor Baker, Winners of In Good Company Challenge," MIT News, Dec. 26, 2018, https://news.mit.edu/2018/mit-agelab-hosts-governor-baker-in-good-company-challenge-winners-1226.

50. Smiley, "What Happens When We Let Tech Care for Our Aging Parents."

51. Massimo Mazzotti, "Algorithmic Life," *Los Angeles Review of Books*, Jan. 22, 2017, https://lareviewofbooks.org/article/algorithmic-life/.

52. Mazzotti, "Algorithmic Life."

53. Mazzotti, "Algorithmic Life."

54. Topol, *Deep Medicine*, 158–59.

55. Topol, *Deep Medicine*, 181.

56. Amos Tversky and Daniel Kahneman, "Judgement under Uncertainty: Heuristics and Biases," *Science* 185, no. 4157 (1974): 1124–231.

57. Christopher Chabris and Daniel Simons, *The Invisible Gorilla: How Our Intuitions Deceive Us* (New York: Broadway Paperbacks, 2009).

58. Topol, *Deep Medicine*, 116–17.

59. Topol, *Deep Medicine*, 139.

60. Kleinman, *The Illness Narratives*, 10.

Chapter Three

Peril

In his Protagoras (380 BC), Plato gives an account of the two Titans Prometheus, meaning "forethought," and his younger brother Epimetheus, which means "after-thought," in their distribution of character traits to the first animals and humans.[1] Epimetheus, true to his name, lacking foresight, first doled out abilities of speed, strength, instinct, keen senses, and camouflage to the animals. When it came to the humans, he had little left. Prometheus inspected his brother's work and realized humans lacked the skills to survive. Greek legend tells us that Prometheus then stole fire from the gods, a theft for which, as we know, he was gruesomely punished. Yet thanks to Prometheus, his theft bestowed upon humans the gifts of reason, speech, the capacity to make tools, and creative inventiveness for technology and art. In Plato's account, Zeus later gave humans notions of justice so that they could live together respectfully in communities.

The poet Hesiod, in two version, his Theogony and his Works and Days (c. 700 B.C.), writes that Zeus punished mortals as well. He ordered his divine craftsman Hephaestus to fashion a snare—a beautiful artificial woman made from earth and water, humanlike in appearance and behavior, Pandora, whose name means "all-encompassing gift" since gods and goddesses bestowed upon her an abundance of talents. In Hesiod's plainly misogynist rendering, Pandora, a kalon kakon, or "beautiful evil," is Zeus' punishment to humans.[2] But the one at fault is not Pandora, the artificial human, a pawn in Zeus' wrath against Prometheus. Epimetheus, again true to his name, did not learn his lesson. Even after Prometheus warned him to not accept gifts from the gods, Epimetheus, so enticed by Pandora, was convinced she was a human and fell for the ruse. We know the rest of the story. Pandora innocently opens the lid to a special jar, pithos, from which afflictions and evils escape, except for one spirit. She closed the lid in time to seal in Hope, elpis.

The meaning behind Pandora sealing in hope remains a mystery. Is hope our only ally, a remedy for suffering? Or is it, trapped in the jar, an affliction we helplessly cling to, a blind hope? Does the jar imprison hope or safeguard us with it?

Spike Jonze's 2013 film "Her" is about an insecure and lonely writer, Theodore Twombly (played by Joaquin Phoenix), who purchases an artificially intelligent operating system, OS1, that he names Samantha. Through powering up the OS1 onto his computer, he can carry "her" anywhere and hear her voice (Scarlett Johansson's) through his earpiece. He can also carry his handheld device enabling her to look out at his world. Growing increasingly obsessed with her, Theodore gradually falls in love with her. As Samantha steadily acquires a 'sense of self'—remember, this is Hollywood—Theodore loses his identity in Samantha, culminating in their cyber-sexual "lovemaking."

Irrespective of the movie's hype and fiction, the story raises a profound question: Is the relationship between Theodore and Samantha real? Our instinctive response: "Of course not! Theodore is a human and Samantha is a machine." But then, what makes the human-to-human encounter any more genuine? Humans fake a lot of things including interest, concern, caring, love, and orgasms. In the future, will these machines not only replace humans but supersede them in the relationship department? Does our infatuation with our current devices embody what philosopher Jean Baudrillard calls the realm of the "hyperreal" in which the machine outreals the real? Regardless of their seduction, certain films capture splinters of truth about human nature. Plato's legendary Allegory of the Cave, one of the earliest 'films,' in Book VII of his *Republic*, describes prisoners in an underground cave who mistake shadows on the wall with reality, confounding what is superficial for truth. Now, with our immersion with the screen and fascination with simulation, we have somehow tickled ourselves into a strange urge, what MIT's Sociology and Personality Psychologist Sherry Turkle in her *Alone Together* calls our "robotic moment."[3] We are at a point in time when we many of us actually *desire* the companionship of our devices over living humans, like humans being drawn more to therapy with chatbots than with other humans.

We described how our human-machine interface radically expresses itself through caring robots. As Shannon Vallor explains, these "carebots" are "designed for use in home, hospital, or other settings to assist in, support, or provide care for the sick, disabled, young, elderly or otherwise vulnerable persons."[4] This combination of artificial intelligence (AI), sensor technology, and robotics for healthcare is a marriage with technology that shows great promise. It is also a dangerous lure, the inevitable consequence of a culture that settles for substitutes. Like Theodore's infatuation with Samantha, caring robots can become our generic drug for human-to-human, flesh-to-flesh contact, for the real thing. But they cannot replace human caregiving. Nor can we have a real conversation with machines. Nonetheless, will robots in fields that require human interaction and dialogue, such as teachers, therapists, coaches, and bartenders like the ones serving drinks now in Las Vegas be enough? Will robots simply be another family member, like Jibo, the brainchild of MIT's Cynthia Breazeal, director of the Media Lab's Personal Robots Group and author of the early trailblazing *Designing Sociable Robots*?[5] We have long had human-machine interaction. However, despite the comfort that machines may offer, they lack the flesh-and-blood touch and embrace we get from a living being. Can we have a true relationship with a caring robot?[6]

IN SEARCH OF MAGIC BULLETS

Robots are extraordinarily useful. They perform tedious and dangerous tasks. Robotic surgery in the future will likely be performed on patients in one country via remote monitoring and skill from a physician abroad. In times of lethal contagion, they are life-saving. Caring robots can enhance interaction among humans where it is badly needed, as in elder care facilities. They can also help human caregivers who encounter more burn-out and stress. By helping out with routine chores, these bots can allow caregivers to spend more time with those they should be caring for. Are they our magic bullet?

The term "magic bullet" originated in medicine. In 1907 German biochemist and Nobel Laureate Paul Ehrlich coined the term in reference to the drug Salvarsan. He found the agent to be effective in treating syphilis, hoping it to be the ideal treatment, a "magic bullet" targeting only pathological organisms responsible for the disease and not adversely affecting anything else. It was aimed to be lesion specific, without collateral damage.[7] No 'friendly fire.' However, with side effects like liver disease and other disorders, Salvarsan was no magic bullet. No doubt, technology has muscle, as internal medicine physician Eric Cassell accurately notes: "I limit the term *technology* to modalities and instrumentalities that greatly extend the power of human action, sensation, or thought independently of their user."[8] And still, the notion prevails among many of us that certain medical technologies and sophisticated digital systems are our magic bullet. Here is an account of a case chronicled by University of California San Francisco (UCSF) Professor of Medicine Robert Wachter in his *The Digital Doctor*. When UCSF installed its new electronic medical system, it had good reason. As in many hospitals prior to the use of electronic medical records, there were abundant medication errors due to human oversight, cumbersome paperwork, faulty communication, wrong records, and the fact that medical personnel were increasingly overwhelmed by systemic demands. Back in 2007, when nearly 200 deaths occurred daily from medical error, many of these were from computer flaws.

As Google research director Peter Norvig asserts, "It's safe to say that every two or three months we have the equivalent of a 9/11 in numbers of deaths due to computer error and medical process."[9] Improved systems and skilled use of electronic medical records was medicine's new magic bullet. It would enable quicker, convenient, cost-saving, and more efficient transfer of medical information to enhance patient outcomes. But, as with Ehrlich's "magic bullet," there were still adverse outcomes. The following is a synopsis of a case based on Wachter's detailed account.[10]

The Over-the-Top Overdose

NEMO (nuclear factor-kappa B essential modulator) syndrome is a rare genetic disorder that results in multiple complications including ongoing infections, abnormal digestion, and bowel ailments. Patients need constant monitoring and a strict regimen of antibiotics to fight infection. In July 2013, a 16-year-old male patient with NEMO was admitted to UCSF Medical Center for a routine colonoscopy. His two brothers had the same disorder. One of them died earlier from the disease.

Weakened from the disease, the teen weighed in at 85 lbs., or 38.5 kg. He needed to be given a proper dose of the antibiotic drug Septra, or trimethoprim. For pediatric patients under 40 kg, the new system was programmed to render medication dosage as mg/kg, milligrams per kilogram. 160 mg of Septra was been the patient's daily intake. That translates to nearly 4.2 mg/kg for the teen. However, due to a string of oversights, bad screen design, lack of human-to-human communication, and blind trust in the system, the computer entry order, programmed to render medication dosage as mg/kg issued his dosage as 160mg/kg, totaling 6,160 mg! His normal daily dosage of 160 mg was increased 38.5 times. Equally alarming, despite this bizarre amount, the night-shift nurse still gave him the pills. Soon after taking them in handfuls and swallowing them, the teen blacked out, suffered a grand mal seizure, and stopped breathing. A Code Blue team arrived just in time to revive him.[11]

What happened? Wachter neatly breaks the case down in order of sequential factors: computer screen design and mode error, incessant alarms, a pharmacy-technician robot, waves of rationalization, and, most important, uncritical, blind trust in the system, program, and machine.

First, *screen design and mode error*. How did the computerized order entry end up entering the dosage as 6,160 mg, 38.5 times the normal dosage? Since the system required weight-based dosing for patients under a certain weight, the pediatric resident assigned to the young man's case carefully noted both dosage and weight on the computer screen. She then sent it electronically to the pediatric clinical pharmacist to sign off on the medication before delivering it to the patient. A reasoned system of checks and balances. Because the *calculated* dose as the resident correctly inscribed it slightly superseded the programmed dose of 160 mg, the pharmacist could not approve until the resident specifically indicated 160 mg as *correct*, which she did by dutifully typing in 160 mg in the computer screen's selected "dose" box and re-sent it to the pharmacist. Right moves so far. But here is the rub, what is called a "mode error" in computer talk.[12] The new system is instructed to have the screen automatically default to the setting when the page was *last visited*. This happens to us when we unintentionally keep the Num Lock or Caps Lock or Insert keys left on for the keyboard. Moreover, on the screen the "order method" box is separate from the "dose" box, enabling the user to set the dosage order either in milligrams or in milligrams per kilograms. *The box was still set at milligrams per kilograms, or mg/kg.* Due to poor screen design and a tight schedule, the resident did not notice this. She filled in the "dose" box correctly to 160 mg, but did not change the "order method" box simply to milligrams which would have amounted to 160 milligrams, the correct dosage. Wrong move. Instead, the order was set for 160 mg/kg *as calibrated*. And the teen weighed 38.5 kg.

Next, *endemic alarms*. Seconds later, the pharmacist received the order. Though alerts popped up on both the resident's and pharmacist's screens, they both clicked off the alarms. Why? Alerts occur chronically in hospitals, most of them false. Alerts happen so often that caregivers can easily experience alarm fatigue. Wachter cites a study by nursing professor Barbara Drew who monitored the number of bedside cardiac alerts over a month in five UCSF's intensive care units.[13] These were just alerts at the bedside (heart rate, EKG, blood pressure, respiration, oxygen), not alarms from IVs or computer systems. Drew's study monitored sixty-six patients daily. She found that each day there were around 187 alerts per patient bed. Wachter sums up her research and adds rates from other alerts:

> Every day, there were about 15,000 alarms across all ICU beds. For the entire month, there were 381,560 alarms across all the five ICUs . . . And those are just the audible ones. If you add the inaudible alerts, those that signal with flashing lights and text-based messages, there were 2,507,822 unique alarms in one month in our ICUs, *the overwhelming majority of them false.*[4] (author emphasis)

Why so many bedside, ICU, and medication alarms? First and foremost, for patients' safety. In addition, built-in alarms protect device manufacturers from litigation. With more than enough on caregivers' plates, not only taking care of patients but spending much of their days filling out their electronic forms, alarm fatigue predictably kicks in. Alarms are often considered to be the usual nuisance alerts.

Third, we come to the *pharmacy-technician robot*. Once the pharmacist signed off, a 7 million dollar Swiss-made pharmacy-technician robot (without a human face, at least not yet) received the order for 160 mg/kg. The teen weighed 38.5 kg. *As programmed*, it methodically selected and counted out the "proper" number of pills, equaling 6,160 mg, sealed them in barcoded packets, and sent them to the patients' floor.[15] The robot is another magic bullet, for good reason. It eliminates the potential for human error in obtaining and measuring the right amount of pills. Plus, the robot works around the clock without grumbling and complaining. No need for breaks or health benefits.

Fourth, *rationalizations*. At first, the night-shift nurse who would distribute the medication, a "floater" who usually worked in the ICU, was stunned by the amount of pills. But rationalizations soon kicked in. Since this is a research hospital, this could be a complex case requiring so many pills. And the pills may be diluted. So she reasoned. She ruled out consulting her charge nurse as this might cause undue interruption. On a busy floor where caregivers are usually under the pressure of time with patients' lives at stake, unnecessary interruptions can sometimes be lethal. There is a clear relationship between interruptions and medication and other clinical errors. According to one study, unnecessary interruptions cause a 12.7 percent increase in clinical errors.[16] Another study focusing on ICU nurses found that they are interrupted every 5 minutes, particularly when involved in high-risk tasks such as administering medication.[17]

Fifth, *blind trust in the program*. Here is the deadliest rationalization: Since the order made it this far, it must have legitimately passed the string of human, computer, algorithm, and barcode checkpoints. The nurse placed a near-blind trust in the system, relying less on her instincts than on the program. Uncritical trust in the program is the weakest link in this chain of human-machine interface. This is where we need to exercise more than ever our critical thinking and trust our senses. This is clearly our major challenge in our interface with machines, particularly in healthcare. As technology and culture author Nicholas Carr points out, blind trust in the program is born out of two cognitive traps: automation complacency and automation bias, similar in effect. Automation complacency helps explain how, amid relentless alarms, health professionals continue to view most of them as nuisance alarms. Carr writes:

> Automation complacency takes hold when a computer lulls us into a false sense of security. We become so confident that the machine will work flawlessly, handling any challenge that may arise, that we allow our attention to drift. We disengage from our work, or at least from a part of it that the software is handling, and as a result may miss signals that something is amiss.[18]

Consider how automation complacency can set us up for unanticipated danger if we slip into the same illusion of total safety and security with caring robots. As for automation bias, it is a major factor driving the nurse's need to rationalize that the strange medication order must be correct. As Carr states, automation bias "creeps in when people give undue weight to the information coming through their monitors. Even when the information is wrong or misleading, they believe it. Their trust in the software becomes so strong that they ignore or discount other sources of information, *including their own senses.*"[19] (author emphasis)

THE ALLURE

Why are we so drawn to certain medical technologies as if they were healthcare's magic bullet? What is their lure? The answer has to do not only with the technologies. It concerns how we relate to them. Technologies fill many of our fundamental needs. Think of the life-saving benefits from radiology, blood tests, CT scans, MRIs, and the numerous benefits of caring robots. All this occurs in the cultural context of our longstanding philosophical ethos of pragmatism. Our intellectual heritage is so deeply pragmatic we associate value with usefulness. An object has value if it is functional and applicable. Sadly, this pertains to living beings as well, hence the plight of elders, finding themselves irrelevant in a society that sets great store by usefulness. This endemic pragmatism has spawned a "technological imperative,"[20] of which the logic is the following: since the only value of a tool or device lies in its applicability, and *because* we have the tools and technologies, for example MRI machines, we feel duty-bound to use them. *Can* implies *should*, a tyranny of technique. There is no more glaring illustration of this technological imperative than in American medicine's flagrant overuse of medical technologies. Yet a tool's maximal use is significantly different from its optimal use. We can assert the same for caring robots.

Here are some key reasons why we are drawn to our technologies. As a start, there is the perpetual lure of the cutting edge. We are naturally drawn to the new. Novelty casts a certain spell on us, and we tend to cast aside the old as useless. We also relish immediate responses and answers. Ours is a society drawn to the quick fix. In addition, we desire certainty and avoid ambiguity and uncertainty. We dread the unknown. And, being *homo faber*, through our technologies we desire to extend our capacity and power. Like Daedalus, we are natural toolmakers. As physicist Max Tegmark puts it in his *Life 3.0*, through our inner software of knowledge and creativity, we can free ourselves from being determined by our biological hardware, a stage he terms "Life 2.0."[21] We will unpack some of these lures, namely the lure of the immediate and quick-fix that technologies offer; the erasure of uncertainty that inherently exists in human-to-human interaction; and the lure of control when certain technologies offer us an illusion of power. The irony, however, is that with all of these, in effect, we stand in peril of deferring authority to our machines. In the case of carebots, 1) the quick, efficient, and safe fix they present in caregiving, particularly in these and future times of contagion, 2) the expectation that they will unambiguously tackle those uncertain and messy caregiving tasks, and 3) the illusion that, due to them, we can control our precarious situation—all these factors contribute to our bestowing authority and deference to carebots and investing blind, uncritical trust in them. Their appeal is deceptive. As in the case above regarding blind faith in electronic health records, they empower users while, at the same time, distancing and disconnecting users from the patient. And with carebots, those who are cared-for may experience a connection, but not the kind of connection with a real flesh-and-blood human.

Immediacy and Quick Fix

Immediacy carries its own spell. We seek fast and ready cures and remedies to be healthy, lose weight, be more sexually active, restore hair, get rid of wrinkles, look younger, be rid of social anxieties, quit smoking, boost athletic performance, etc. This is most apparent as we transmute routine yet undesirable features of life, including aging and death, into pathologies. Before its fall from grace, part of the popularity of the former wonder-drug Prozac (fluoxetine) rested on public perception that it relieved us not only from clinical depression but also from life's minor distresses. Consider the lab results, scan reports, and other tallies from the cornucopia of tests we take as patients. The value of these tests is unquestionable. Having a routine physical is all-important. Having my six-month CT scans after chemotherapy were undeniably vital. While they naturally incurred some anxiety, with good results they offered reassurance. Our tests are often no doubt necessary as they manifest the driving force of medical science, science we never abandon, but only develop further. These tests carry an immediacy. At the same time their immediacy unhinges context.[22]

There is a world of difference between *content* and *context*. Relying on content and ignoring context is perilous. Philosopher Martha Nussbaum addresses this when she probes matters pertaining to caring for the disabled, strongly insisting on the importance of context. Her "capability approach" to caring means that the kind of care we offer depends upon the *circumstances of who is cared-for*, whether they are children, elders, disabled persons, etc. At the same time, though their needs differ, caring always aims to protect and maintain their safety and dignity. Moreover, the quality of caring is wide since it indelibly affects all those related to the persons being cared-for.[23] However, in the medical world, content often wins out over context, a bias toward measurability that rules throughout our society.[24] Hence, another magic bullet—data. Data tells it like it is. No need for knowing the patient's culture, beliefs, past, values, interests, desires, or fears—the patient's context.

A steady, soundless, metronome beats among immediacy, speed, distance, and forgetfulness, further disconnecting caregiving from those being cared-for. Our culture is obsessed with speed, getting from A to C in the quickest way possible. Look at the way we drive, always in a rush, in a hurry to get to our jobs where we will spend the next eight hours or more. In his brilliant novel *Slowness*, Milan Kundera writes "Speed is the form of ecstasy the technical revolution has bestowed on man."[25] Our newest laptops boast faster Internet speed. Our medical theater of the Absurd: under institutional pressure, physicians have so many patients to see in a day; patients arrive on time for their appointments and then wait it out to finally meet with their doctor for, on average, seven minutes. Fixated with speed and immediate results, we cut ourselves off from time's natural flow, its gravity. This is not the speed of sprinters. For the sprinter, each moment of the race flows with body and mind in sync. This is the speed of machines the human has created, and "from then on, his own body is outside the process, and he gives over to a speed that is noncorporeal, nonmaterial, pure speed, speed itself, ecstasy speed."[26] This kind of speed breeds distance—geographic, physical, cognitive, emotional. It is a distance that slices away the precious context of past-present-future, linked movements in a symphony. Speed produces forgetfulness. Slowing down enables memory. For Kundera, it comes down to a clear-cut formula, an "existential mathematics": "the degree of slowness is directly proportional to the intensity of memory; the degree of speed in directly proportional to the intensity of forgetting."[27]

Apply this to caring robots. Caring robots have a vital instrumental, practical, and life-saving value. Japan's robot RIBA II (Robot for Interactive Body Assistance) can lift patients and help prevent back injuries to nurses and orderlies. Lifting patients also helps to abate a patient's painful bedsores. We pointed out earlier how Japan's aging population compels the push to design caring robots for elders. The country's shocking rate of seniors over 65, predicted to reach over 40 percent by 2050, is not the only driving force. Japan has a steadily declining birth rate. In addition, because less native citizens are entering the caregiving profession, more immigrants seek to become household partners and companions for elders. With an increasing numbers of *gaijin* (foreigners) in caregiving roles, robots are a way to help soothe anxieties many Japanese elders may have with foreign caretakers. Moreover, by having more robots caring for seniors, the hope is that this can free up more women, the typical caregivers, to marry, have children, and help restore a declining birthrate. Here we have a clear example of viewing technology as an efficient "fix" to address deeper sociocultural problems that are remnants of endemic xenophobia and sexism.[28]

Painting with a broader brush and using a utilitarian litmus test, consider another set of possible long-range consequences. In stressing the crucial need for human-to-human contact, Brazilian philosopher Darlei Dall'Agnol points out,

> Given the present stage in the development of robotics and the idea of respectful care, we must not regard robots as substitutes for human carers. It seems that a human and perhaps in the future a sensible artificial person must always be in the loop of care supervising robot caregivers . . . Consequently, current robots may help, but they cannot be seen as the definite solution for the problem of social exclusion of the elderly.[29]

Aside from the vagueness of "sensible artificial person," the last point is particularly insightful—"social exclusion of the elderly." *Will there be a time when human caregivers willingly pass the baton of caregiving on to machines?* Currently, more families are increasingly fragmented with family members distanced from each other and from their communities. Connectivity via devices is certainly one way to stay in touch. How we have interacted with each other during our COVID-19 pandemic is proof. For that these devices have become invaluable. But, as I maintain throughout, *connectivity is not connectedness*. Connectedness in the fullest sense demands physical, embodied interaction and presence. Will we eventually give our blessing to having a robot, even one with "super intelligence" and self-consciousness, take care of grandpa? Will we then take his being *cared for* and *cared about* for granted? This could offer us a reasonable "out," an excuse to evade or diminish our personal, familial, and indeed moral responsibility to be with grandpa as well as we can. Like the night-shift nurse distributing the massive medication dosage to the patient, will we continue to trust the program and the machine? *Will trusting blindly that his "caregiver" will take good care of him become our default posture?* How far are we willing to trust the system? Now is the time to urgently ponder these questions, particularly in a social climate sponged in individualism carried to its extreme and increasing unashamed narcissism.

Erasing Uncertainty

There is the joke about the man who, tipsy after a few drinks, loses his car keys at night in a parking lot. He tells this to a policeman while he continues to look for his keys under the parking lot light. The policeman asks if he lost his keys near the light, and the man replies, "No, but the light is much better here." Diagnostic tools can sometimes be the night light. In other words, tests produce concrete and specific data that in turn legitimizes a treatment strategy, or why the man searches under the light. A patient's testimony does not offer the same degree of validation. A patient complains of chronic pain. Chronic headaches. Sleeplessness. Yet because tests show no abnormalities, they invalidate the complaint. Relying on technologies while minimizing the patient's own account and lived experience shifts the question. All this amounts to a significant disconnect and distancing from the patient's singularity. We have transformed the real patient into an "iPatient," coined by Abraham Verghese to refer to the patient pared down to data from tests.[30] The iPatient is the patient quantified, the patient *defined* by tests. The iPatient is not the real patient, a person with lived experience with illness in real time. With real patients, there is ambiguity and uncertainty. Nonetheless, says Cassell, "physicians mistakenly believe they can reduce uncertainty by changing the patient's problem to one for which there is a technological answer. They then reduce the problem from that of the patient to that of an organ or part for which a technology exists, and they *distance themselves from the patient by employing that technology*"[31] (author emphasis).

Medical knowledge carries uncertainty, and ambiguity can be perplexing. This is the challenge for medical students upon entering the noble calling of medicine, noble because it delicately interweaves science and humanity in striving to alleviate suffering. And the distinctive lure of medical technologies lies in their erasure of real-life, human nuance. As we continue in American healthcare to tout our sophisticated medical tools, the more seized we are by the illusion of certainty. "Sophistication" is the operative term here. Cassell sees a different meaning of "sophisticated" when it comes to technologies: "the development of sophistication in nontechnological pursuits involves appreciation of complexity and ambiguity. Sophistication in technology, I believe, goes in the other direction. More sophistication means less ambiguity; the better the equipment, the clearer the values."[32] He cites the case of an asymptomatic middle-aged man who wants to join a fitness program. He first checks with his cardiologist who suggests he undergo a series of tests—treadmill, stress, and coronary arteriogram. The arteriogram reveals atherosclerosis. Because atherosclerosis is technically coronary heart disease, he submits to coronary artery angioplasty, or percutaneous coronary intervention (PCI), an invasive procedure. Cassell points out that there is little evidence in the current literature that shows positive results either with or without the procedure.[33] In a recent *Lancet* article, researchers reported that "In patients with medically treated angina and severe coronary stenosis, PCI did not increase exercise time by more than the effect of a placebo procedure. The efficacy of invasive procedures can be assessed with a placebo control, as is standard for pharmacotherapy."[34] Yet tests and procedures aid in erasing ambiguity.

We are drawn to what we know for certain. And what is certain is on the screen from test and lab results. Numbers don't lie. Neither do they tell the whole truth. We realize this only when we can get a glint of the real patient, who is an ongoing story, an intimate narrative that cannot be quantified, measured, nor captured on the screen. Caring for the patient means connecting with the patient. It means taking one's eyes off the screen and looking at and speaking directly *with*, not *to*, the patient. It demands eye contact.[35] We learn the immeasurable value of eye contact from early on. A good deal of our emotional and social stability comes from interactions with others through eye contact. Eye contact is a vital ingredient in building a ladder to empathy, healthcare's most important virtue. In their work on the relation between eye contact and brain activity, cognitive scientists Atsushi Senju and Mark Johnson examine how eye contact stimulates the brain's subcortical routes. Such activation "modulates key structures involved in the cortical social brain network." All this affects how we process facial expressions including smiles.[36] This direct correlation between eye contact and brain activity enables connecting with another's feelings, a neural basis for empathy. How often does your doctor actually look at you? *Even when he looks at you does he see you?* His laptop can shield him from unscripted conversation, one in which you can sense whether he is present, there *with* you and *for* you.

Caring robots act in ways that help erase uncertainties and ambiguities in caring for another. In a sense, they act as a caregiving "decision support tool" (DST) upon which we can rely when it comes to caring. But, like the case earlier concerning electronic health records, blind trust in the system leads to adverse consequences. So also with uncritical trust in DSTs. Social scientists Batya Friedman and Peter Khan foresaw this precarious reliance in 1992 regarding the computer-based system APACHE (Acute Physiology and Chronic Health Evaluation) to help ascertain prognoses for patients in critical care and in ICUs, even determining when life-support for patients in ICUs might be appropriately withdrawn. Their account of undue dependency on the DST of APACHE, since then upgraded, as a computer generated decision tool in intensive care units raises red flags about physician deference to the system. They assert that "it may become the practice of critical care staff to act on APACHE's recommendations somewhat automatically, and increasingly difficult for even an experienced physician to challenge the 'authority' of APACHE's recommendation, since to challenge APACHE would be to challenge the medical community."[37] It becomes a dicey situation for patients when "computer prediction dictates clinical decision."[38] When we consider the panoply of caring's "soft" issues such as respecting a patient's self-determination, the role of family and web of relations, patient values, beliefs regarding "quality-of-life," and cultural worldviews, relying solely on "hard" algorithm-derived decisions by machines abrogates our own moral, caring responsibility.

By placing too much trust in the system, whether electronic medical records or the APACHE system used in ICUs, we evidence adverse, sometimes fatal, consequences. In much the same way, we can place blind trust in our caring robots. The more effective carebots become in ensuring safety for patients, elders, bedridden, disabled, and other vulnerable persons, the more easily we trust their efficacy to the point where they become crutches for our own obligations. Families may defer more to the carebot. Can we confidently claim that "Grandma is in good hands"? Even better hands?

The Power Delusion

Medical technologies offer control in circumstances of uncertainty and ambiguity. Control is a matter of knowledge, Prometheus' gift to humans, not brute force. Digging further, there is a deeper motive at play—power over our most human frailty, our mortality, the worm in the apple. The penalty for defying Yahweh's (or Elohim's) command to not eat the fruit of the tree of knowledge of good and evil included expulsion from the Garden, permanent unattainability of utopia, and condemnation to a life of toil and pain, finally ending in death. But the real sentence is that we *know* we will die. Mortality is not the curse. The blight lies in knowing that death awaits us, an awareness that ultimately saps our sense of control and power. The cold certainty of death is so unsettling, at least throughout much of Western culture, we make efforts to hide it, deny, even alter it. In his brilliant *The Denial of Death*, Ernest Becker terms this our "impossible paradox": "The ever-present fear of death in the normal biological functioning of our instinct of self-preservation, as well as our utter obliviousness to this fear in our conscious life."[39]

The gifted artist Michael Ayrton, whose sculpture of Icarus III graces London's Old Change Court, was gripped by the legend of Daedalus and Icarus. His novel *The Maze Maker* is Daedalus' first-person account of his life.

> My name is Daedalus and I am a technician. This I chose to be. I have made many things in many places and done so cunningly, for that is the meaning of my name. I have constructed buildings and planned fortifications. I am proficient in stone carving and I can make the forms of gods in wood, completely joined. I have made many tools to do these things and invented others to make the work simpler and have it better done. Also I can paint images and I am adept at mechanical contrivance. All these things I can do as well as any other, be he who he may.[40]

Technology is all too-human. Daedalus reincarnated, we are tool makers. Yet our obsession with our tools whereby we become tools of our tools, slaves of our creations, is, at its bedrock, a consequence of our desire to overcome death. As much as we try to postpone aging and death, they still pay us a visit. Max Tegmark writes, "Yet despite the most powerful technologies we have today, all life forms we know of remain fundamentally limited by their biological hardware."[41] Indeed, having robots with more humanlike appearances, like a human face, will likely reignite our entrenched angst about our own mortality. Our denial of death may shape any enthusiasm we have regarding carebots with human faces.

We humans need to believe we are in control, particularly during the dire circumstances of uncertainty, high risk, and unpredictability of our prolonged COVID-19 crisis. Thankfully, after painstaking nonstop research, much of it using robotics, we have developed effective vaccines. Yet with machines, how much control are we willing to cede? How willing are we to rely on autonomous machines? Given the ubiquity of technologies in our lives, there is always a tension between our sense of freely chosen self-determination and our constant reliance on the tools we choose and ones chosen for us.

Though we take their work for granted, attending to the product rather than what goes into it, designers play a crucial role in all this. We largely assume some zone of dull neutrality in behind-the-scenes expertise, impartial technical wizardry. However, designers *design*. Absent intent and malice, they unavoidably and unknowingly imbed their views as to the scope, degree, and nature of the interaction users will have with their devices. Designers of carebots aim to develop a caring machine through enabling certain caring tasks. In doing so, they design the *kinds* of interaction with human users. We are being designed as well as the machine. It is subtly happening through what we can call the "rule of switch," which rests upon the premise that we humans need to relate to others. The less we interact with each other, the more we switch allegiances, in this case, to a machine. And the more we engage with our machines, our devices, our screens—all nonliving, non-spirited, dead objects—the less we feel a need to interact with other humans. As philosopher Blay Whitby pointedly asserts, the market for technologies such as robots for love and sex (à la David Levy's firestorm prediction in his *Love and Sex with Robots* that in the near future we will come to desire intimate relationships with robots) thrives in the absence of human-to-human connection. "In blunt terms: if everybody chose a human lover, the market for robot lovers would be very small. The market for robot lovers and other caring technologies is maximized in the situation where nobody chooses human companionship."[42] The setting for caring robots is ripe. We are primed.

Enter the As-If World

Have you been in the company of those who act as if they are really speaking with our ever-popular "Siri" or "Alexa," for instance about the weather? If I ask Alexa about the meaning of happiness does "she" understand the question? Or "Hey, Siri, does God exist?" Will Siri be discerning enough to respond, "Michael, I cannot properly answer your question unless you first tell me what *your* idea of God is." Alexa and Siri may act *as if* they know, but acting and knowing are not the same. As Sherry Turkle reminds us in her ever-timely *Reclaiming Conversation*, the seduction of the "as if" is real. Influenced by the psychoanalyst Helene Deutsch's landmark study of the "as-if personality," Turkle raises pivotal concerns regarding our human-machine interface.[43] Turkle hits a crucial vein, underscoring throughout her work that a machine can act "as if" it understands and "as if" it cares. Caring robots, in marvelously sophisticated ways, are designed to perform *as if* they really care. Max Tegmark admits the possibility of AI becoming upgraded enough to create better AI by itself without human intervention. For instance, Google's DeepMind team developed the AI system AlphaZero that, after learning on its own, surpassed its AI predecessor AlphaGo, not only defeating it in the highly complex ancient Chinese strategic game of Go but becoming the world's number one chess program.[44] On its own, such highly advanced AI system can perform "as if" it can exceed any level of human intelligence and creativity. Yet whether the system genuinely *understands* what it is doing is another matter. Tegmark highlights this in AI language processing.

> From being trained on massive data sets, it discovers patterns and relations involving words without ever relating these words to anything in the real world … It may then conclude from this [patterns and relations] that the difference between "king" and "queen" is similar to that between "husband" and "wife"—but it still has no clue what it is to be male or female. Or even that there is such a thing as a physical reality out there with space, time and matter.[45]

The world of simulation is the world of "as if." It is a world of pretense, as when we don our Halloween costumes to look "as if" we are ghouls, or when an actress impeccably and convincingly acts "as if" she is Lady Macbeth. In the world of acting, performance is everything.[46] Surely, for the duration of the play, behaving like Lady Macbeth requires *being* Lady Macbeth. Great actors live their roles and become their characters. Until the curtain closes.

We have always anthropomorphized inanimate objects. The more we feel some sort of bond, the more we bestow human qualities, even human names. A 1944 classic study demonstrated how subjects described the movement of geometric figures as if they were human.[47] We assign humanness to toys, dolls, automobiles, boats, etc. I motorcycled throughout Europe on my BSA that I named Kriemhilde after my German friend in Hamburg. And I always biked with my trusty Gibson guitar Sue. We choose the type of voice that gives us directions in our auto's GPS. I prefer the soft, female one with a slight accent. We anthropomorphize our pets, even robotic pets like Paro, and like Jim who calls his CareCoach puppy avatar Pony. What is odd about all this, however, is that even when we *know* that the machine does not really listen, know, and understand what we feel, we are still drawn to interrelate with it. We surrender to the performance, what Turkle labels the "ELIZA Effect," named after computer scientist Joseph Weizenbaum's popular computer program that simulates responses typically given by a Rogerian psychotherapist. Many, like this young man talking with a robot, still want to "feel in the presence of a knowing other that cares about them." Turkle describes his interaction: "A young man, twenty-six, talks with a robot named Kismet that makes eye contact, reads facial expressions, and vocalizes with the cadences of human speech. The man finds Kismet so supportive that he speaks with it about the ups and downs of his day."[48] In this early prototype, the robot Kismet simulates autonomous response to humans' facial cues *as if* it was authentically interacting, displaying various emotional states such as anger, fear, sadness, interest, and responding to cues like tone of voice and pauses in order to avoid interrupting. Kismet, one of the early "social robots" featured in Cynthia Breazeal's pioneering work, is now displayed in the MIT Museum. Breazeal's is a groundbreaking attempt at programming robots *as if* they can genuinely interact with humans.[49] What is endlessly fascinating is how we respond to these machines, like nursing home residents bonding with the baby harp seal Paro as if Paro was their own pet, or a substitute for their child or grandchild.

Aside from the implicit deception in marketing "sociable robots," we generally admit that their "humanness" extends only *up to a point*. However, for nursing home residents who are desperate for human contact, particularly with family and friends, who spend their days looking for that door in their room to open, such marketing exploits their emotional needs. Attachments they form with their robot companions are clearly understandable. And carebots come with no strings attached. They will not cheat or steal. They are dependable, without mood swings, always patient. Is this not better than having no contact? At the same time, unquestioning deference to carebots diminishes our moral fiber. It is one thing to know that grandma will be safer through the watchful eyes of her carebot, and that she will be dutifully reminded to take her medications. It is another to rest content, assured that her carebot is all she needs. As political scientist Joan Tronto poignantly asserts, *taking care of* is not the same as *caring for*. In typical fashion, Sherry Turkle's summation is spot-on: "We are built to nurture what we love but also to love what we nurture. *Nurturance turns out to be a 'killer app.' Once we take care of a digital creature or teach or amuse it, we become attached to it, and then behave 'as if' the creature cares for us in return.*"[50]

Carebots clearly fulfill the first two stages of James Moor's categories of artificial moral agents.[51] First, they are "ethical impact agents." This focuses on the moral impact and consequences of their acts. Nursing home residents are delighted to have Paro visit them. They spend their days waiting for someone to see them, to speak with someone who listens to them, someone who is there-for-them. Voilà, Paro. Carebots are also what Moor calls "implicit ethical agents," having to do with their intended design. They are deliberately designed in ways that reliably monitor and enhance residents' safety. In situations of endemic infection, ensuring this safety is all-the-more pressing. Just as remotely operated vehicles (ROVs) are deployed to protect troops while inflicting damage on enemy targets, a riskless engagement, carebots are intended to ensure the safety of both caregivers and those cared-for. Of course, there is a world of difference in context and purpose between ROVs, fighter drones, bomb detectors and disposers, and caring robots. During times of contagion, carebots offer a riskless caring, at least without the risks that come with human caregivers.

Is all this simply a matter of encoding the bot to anticipate a full range of potential events and circumstances and act accordingly, even acting morally *as if* they are moral agents? Carebots are fixed to be reliable, on-call all day and night, without complaint. Yet here is a moral red flag. *Being programmed to act reliably* is not the same as *being* reliable. Carebots have no choice in the matter. *Being* reliable assumes a sufficient degree of moral agency. *Being* dependable means having the freedom to choose to be dependable or not. Carebots act as if they are reliable. Making ethical choices, however—to be or not be reliable, caring, trustworthy, honest, sensitive, attentive, compassionate, etc.—entails being aware of the options and making the choice. Freely making a moral decision means knowing to some degree what is at stake. Yale computer scientist Drew McDermott says it crisp and clear. "The ability to do ethical decision-making . . . requires knowing what an ethical conflict is, i.e., a clash between self-interest and what ethics prescribes."[52] Carebots do not have this clash. Though preset to recognize some types of ethical conflict, they lack the capacity for self-interest. They act as if they are morally sensitive. They act as if they care. Do they?

WHAT IS CARING?

By acting in ways that *demonstrate* caring, carebots embody performance. Is performance sufficient in genuine caring? Performance can signify a moral act without sufficient motive and intent. This is the "functional morality" described more fully by Wendell Wallach and Colin Allen incorporating a degree of autonomy and sensitivity that is not the same as an entity possessing "full moral agency."[53] Though they may have functional morality, caring robots cannot genuinely care. When we examine the nature of caring, unsurprisingly, most of the major voices are women. Most human caregivers, both professional and family, are women. While a current of gender issues course through much of this, we will not inspect them here. For now, here are some brief summaries of views toward caring as a deeply human trait.

Voices from Psychology, Philosophy, and Nursing

The prominent feminist and psychologist Carol Gilligan challenged her professor Lawrence Kohlberg, a leading authority on moral development, arguing that moral decision-making, particularly among females, entails considerations of feelings and relationships, not just utilizing moral principles and rules. Kohlberg, instead, held that understanding and applying moral principles and rules to specific cases were standards of moral maturity that he believed males tend to arrive at before females. Gilligan clearly focuses instead on the bigger picture, arguing that the mere application of principles and duties is short-sighted. Due to her stress on a relational dynamic involving responsibilities, Gilligan sparked further interest in the nature of caring relationships.[54]

Philosopher Nel Noddings takes Gilligan's ideas further, applying them to moral development, maternal care, and education.[55] She systematically develops an ontology of caring as a key attribute in being human, insisting that we are naturally embedded in relationships that pose choices to us to offer care and to be cared for. For Noddings, because of our nature as complex humans with basic human needs, caring is more than simply a matter of performing tasks. Caring, like moral action, is more than just *doing* the right thing. Genuine caring requires *being* good, having the right motives and possessing good character. Her ideas carry a strong Aristotelian flavor since Aristotle emphasized the centrality of becoming a virtuous person through cultivating good character. Simply acting in good ways is not enough. Good character, intent, and motive are equally important, something to think about regarding caring robots. Noddings' insights also come close to Japanese philosopher Watsuji Tetsuro's concept of *aidagara*, or "in-betweenness." Who we are comprises both individuality and relationship. Our *aida*, "in-between," constitutes our lived experience. We each live inherently "in-between," in-between humans, in-between other living creatures, and in-between the natural environment. We inhabit both a natural climate and social climate, and these climates influence who we are and become. Our in-betweenness thereby has profound ontological significance. We are both individual and relational. We intrinsically affect and are affected by others, particularly those close to us at home and work. Swimming in this sea of interdependence, we inescapably bear personal and moral responsibility to others and to the natural world.

We can add to these views the care gestalt offered by Amartya Sen and Martha Nussbaum, who support a capabilities approach to caring. Though not a strictly systematic theory, it underscores the need to enhance human flourishing through healthy interaction with the environment including people and other living beings. In view of this approach's strongly pragmatic orientation, technology enables humans to interface with their surroundings to build and sustain personal well-being. For elders in particular this means questioning whether carebots better empower them through safeguarding basic capabilities like health, control, and bodily integrity.

Caring robots for elders have far-reaching implications for nursing, in essence a caring profession. The American Nurses Association makes this clear from the outset.

> Nursing can be described as both an art and a science; a heart and a mind. At its heart, lies a fundamental respect for human dignity and an intuition for a patient's needs . . . Nursing has a unifying ethos: In assessing a patient, nurses do not just consider test results. Through the critical thinking exemplified in the nursing process . . . nurses use their judgment to integrate objective data with subjective experience of a patient's biological, physical and behavioral needs.[56]

This "unifying ethos" emphasizes that nursing's complex process of assessment, critical thinking, judgment, planning, and implementation is *more than simply a matter of routinely completing tasks*. Foreseeing the impact of robotic technologies in healthcare in 1992, nurse practitioner Mary Lou Peck neatly captures the soul of caring.

> Only a step beyond this is the development of robots who can do a better surgical job than a human being. What is missing from this scenario? Tender loving care. That is the nurse's job, and it is something that computers cannot do because it involves feelings and human communication . . *Human response will never be replaced by technology*, and the unchanging need for the nurses' caring function will assure their future.[57] (author emphasis)

Tender loving care involves embodied human presence, human interaction, and certainly the distinctive human touch. It brings us back to the nature of caring. Caring is our most human act, caring for the whole person, a person with a history and ongoing story. Moreover, caring is a mutual act in which carer and cared-for engage with, appreciate, and affirm each other in unspoken, unassuming ways.[58]

Designing Care?

Instrumental aims are task-oriented. As we have discussed, more is involved in true caring. Ethics consultant on robotics Rosangela Barcaro and others argue that genuine caring is between humans and carries moral weight.

> True caretaking is only possible between and among human persons, since only human relationships have the potential to shape moral decisions in the framework of a mutual relationship between the one-caring and the cared-for . . . Glances, hugs, and silences are among the elements that shape the caring relationship and transmit compassion, participation, happiness or sadness.[59]

But if their value lies strictly in their instrumentality, designing these robots is a matter of crucial significance. Can care be designed? With our fast-moving advances in artificial intelligence (AI), will we reach a point when we can actually design caring? Consider efforts in designing "artificial superintelligence" that aim to surpass human intelligence in ways that enable itself to self-program. Think of a computer that can rewrite its own program. According to engineer John Loeffler, if it thinks on its own in ways that exceed the human mind, getting rid of it once it has gained ground is nearly unachievable. He writes, "with something this intelligent, it could discover ways of preserving itself that we would think completely impossible because we lack the intelligence to know how to accomplish it, like trying to conceive of the physics of an airplane while having the brain capacity of a baboon."[60] Is this something we should fear? Loeffler adds, "An artificial superintelligence then will be what we make of it, just as children are more than just the biological product of their parents, so it's critical that we decide as a civilization just what sort of artificial superintelligence we wish to create."[61]

University of Sheffield cognitive scientist Tony Prescott is working on designing self-conscious humanoid robots he calls iCubs. For Prescott, a critical premise hinges upon thinking of "self" as a process and not some static entity, "a process being a virtual machine running inside a physical one, as when a program runs on a computer."[62] According to Prescott, this "self-consciousness" is able to distinguish itself from others, have a sense of past and future, possess a life story with goals and values, be aware of an inner life, and hopefully be capable of empathy. Prescott describes this in light of brain patterns in mirror neurons.

Your ability to interpret another person's actions using your own body schema is partly down to mirror neurons—cells in your brain that fire both when you perform a given movement and when you see someone else perform it . . . As a result, iCub can rapidly acquire new hand gestures, and learn sequences of actions involved in playing games or solving puzzles, simply by watching people perform these tasks. To achieve empathy will require extending the system further so that iCub recognises and mirrors both the physical (movement) and emotional state of the person being observed.[63]

Can this enormously enhanced 'self-conscious' robot eventually replace human caregivers? The term "conscious," though often used, is a notoriously difficult idea to sufficiently grasp—"consciousness." How a cognitive scientist defines "conscious" can be rather different from how a philosopher characterizes the nature of the human mind. The brain, having over one thousand billion neurons, countless synapses and energy charges of quarks and electrons, can be separate from the mind. Or not. The jury is out, at least among philosophers. Nonetheless, Prescott's aim in this kind of "enhancement" can threaten to fundamentally compromise the trust so essential in forming an authentic, caring relationship. Especially since caring is a dynamic process, not a static event. Philosopher of technology Aimee van Wynsberghe argues likewise.

If, however, the robot is (someday) capable of understanding what it is doing and why, and may act in a skillful manner, the robot still poses a threat to the holistic process of care . . . that care is not one task or a series of tasks but is a compilation of practices to meet the needs of the actors, each practice building on the last.[64]

These "enhancements" of caring robots opens a Pandora's Jar, or Box, with all sorts of philosophical, moral, and legal issues.[65] Will a time come when robotic nurses surpass human nurses such that there will then be alleged "superior" robotic nurses and "inferior" human nurses? Do we consider these robots "persons," assigning them moral status? These questions inevitably generate profound challenges regarding profession, identity, and selfhood.

The Matter of Harm

They also reveal another potential peril from the use of carebots. This is not so much the danger of physical injury, although there is always the potential of a system going awry. Recall Isaac Asimov's Three Laws of Robotics that he wrote back in 1942.[66]

1. A robot may not injure a human being or, through inaction, allow a human being to come to harm.
2. A robot must obey orders given it by human beings except where such orders would conflict with the First Law.
3. A robot must protect its own existence as long as such protection does not conflict with the First or Second Law.

Later on, when he envisioned robots in warfare, Asimov added his "zeroth law" in his 1985 novel *Robots and Empire*: "A robot may not harm humanity, or, by inaction, allow humanity to come to harm."[67] When we apply these laws to carebots, no one of them seem to be violated if we define "harm" strictly in physical terms, as in physical injury or death. Yet, if we broaden "harm" to include emotional, psychological, and social assaults, this opens the door to the potential for harm.[68] There is clear injury when one's privacy is violated even without that person's knowledge of the violation. "Harm" is a double-edged sword, notably in the area of personal privacy. 24/7 monitoring makes perfect sense when an elder heads to the top of the basement stairs, or when pots are boiling on the stove. Yet, while ensuring residents' safety, a 24-hour watch can be intrusive when residents are on the toilet or taking a bath. Will they have some say in their surveillance? And the more autonomous carebots become, the more difficult it will be to monitor the monitoring.

We can come up with a shopping list of unintended possible harms. But some harms run deeper. More for our purposes regarding caring robots, let us add to Asimov's list another—"The three laws of Robo LDK," referring to humans coexisting with robots in their living (including sleeping), dining, and kitchen (LDK) areas, the foremost areas where robots can assist humans.

Law 1. Robots must be useful to humans, and provide protection, *caregiving,* and *attend to their spiritual and psychological needs* (the usefulness principle).
Law 2. Robots must be able to interact with and relate to humans in a reassuring manner (the safety principle).
Law 3. A robot's body conforms to its function and role in the household. As a physical body living in close proximity to humans, robots must be able to exercise Laws 1 and 2.[69] (author emphasis)

These laws were formulated in 2007 when a public contest was held in Japan between roboticists and information technology specialists in various cities to demonstrate human-robot cohabiting, resulting in a guidebook containing the three laws, *Robotto no iru kurashi* (Living with Robots). Many Japanese are already prepped to co-exist with robots, but what is especially striking is the emphasis in the first law on robots' "caregiving" (*iyashi*) and "spiritual and psychological" comfort: "Robots must be useful to humans, and provide protection, caregiving, and attend to their spiritual and psychological needs." One can rightly ask, "What harm is there in grandma having a companion? For her, it makes her feel happy." No doubt, for many nursing home residents, it is a pleasant relief from the suffocating routine of their days. But attachment to carebots can trigger increasing detachment from humans, particularly family and friends. Then again, though not a healthy solution, isn't it better than nothing? Perhaps even better than humans? In other words, what matters is how grandma and grandpa and others feel and behave, not whether their carebot really cares. Can humans themselves feel cared for by their carebots? Human caregivers can cheat, steal, lie, complain, get angry, frustrated, impatient, abusive, and be unreliable and untrustworthy. Sadly, much abuse comes from family members, spouses, and children.

At this point in their design, engineers are clearly working to prevent physical and mechanical malfunctions particularly if they might lead to harm. This is consistent with their professional ethics as engineers. The National Society of Professional Engineers (NSPE) Code of Ethics states that engineers must "hold paramount the safety, health, and welfare of the public."[70] This duty especially carries weight in the dire circumstances of pandemics. There will always be a design challenge, particularly when robots become more autonomous over time. As we will explore more fully in our last chapter, any solution to challenges regarding carebots does not lie simply with the machines themselves. Rather, it involves how we ourselves interact with them. In other words, yes, let us design, if possible, "moral machines," or at least build in those granular patterns that come close to acting, or performing, morally. At the same time we need to reexamine our own roles, relationships, and moral obligations. Any "solution" is necessarily symbiotic. If we simply leave it up to machine design, we then abdicate our own moral duties to those for whom we care, and to each other.

Our Human Folly

If there is anything we can confidently assert throughout our COVID-19 pandemic, it is that we cannot depend on people to behave sensibly and safely. This is hardly new. Human history is a history of human folly. Because we wear seat belts, we can speed. Since we have low-flow showers, we can take longer showers and use up more water. Because we have diet pills, we can eat until we are stuffed. Because we wear masks, we can violate physical distance and be on top of the person in front of us in line. Apply this to nursing home settings. Carebots can be our technological fix, our facemask, our magic bullet for the deeper social and moral issues of human neglect of the marginal and vulnerable.

Carebots offer marvelous benefits, particularly in light of the global shortage of human caregivers. They can relieve stress and fatigue among caregivers and families, address the loneliness of marginal and vulnerable groups, and, in future pandemics, protect human caregivers and the cared-for from infection. Yet relying more on caring robots can bring about less empathy, less human-to-human contact, less face-to-face connecting. Robert Sparrow and Linda Sparrow, who have written extensively on the impact of technologies, remarked presciently in 2006, "it is naïve to think that the development of robots to take over tasks currently performed by humans in caring roles would not lead to a reduction of human contact for those people being cared for."[71] For families, carebots can become their technological crutch, particularly if we have more widespread contagions and their variants forcing lockdowns and social distancing. Human companionship is crucial. Can carebots replace this? Suppose they look more like us? What if they have human faces?

NOTES

1. Here is my rendition of the account, originally found in Plato, *Protagorus*, trans. Benjamin Jowett and ed. Gregory Vlastos (Indianapolis, IN: The Bobbs-Merrill Company, Inc., 1956), sections 320c–322b, 18–20.

2. This is a brief retelling of the Pandora legend. The fuller description is in Adrienne Mayor's superb *Gods and Robots: Myths, Machines, and Ancient Dreams of Technology* (Princeton, NJ: Princeton University Press, 2018), 157–60.

3. Sherry Turkle, *Alone Together: Why We Expect More from Technology and Less from Each Other* (New York: Basic Books, 2011), 3–13.

4. Shannon Vallor, "Carebots and Caregivers: Sustaining the Ethical Ideal of Care in the 21st Century," *Journal of Philosophy and Technology* 24 (2011): 251–68. See also Shannon Vallor, *Technology and the Virtues: A Philosophical Guide to a Future Worth Wanting* (New York: Oxford University Press, 2016), 208–229.

5. Cynthia Breazeal, *Designing Sociable Robots* (Cambridge, MA: MIT Press, 2002).

6. Michael C. Brannigan, "Does Seamus the Robot Care for Me?" *Albany Times Union*, February 27, 2011, https://www.timesunion.com/opinion/article/Does-Seamus-the-robot-care-for-me-1032481.php.

7. Stanley Joel Reiser, *Technological Medicine: The Changing World of Doctors and Patients* (New York: Cambridge University Press, 2009), 187.

8. Eric J. Cassell, *Doctoring: The Nature of Primary Care Medicine* (Oxford: Oxford University Press, 1997), 63.

9. Cited in Wendell Wallach and Colin Allen, *Moral Machines: Teaching Robots Right from Wrong* (New York: Oxford University Press, 2009), 22.

10. Robert Wachter, *The Digital Doctor: Hope, Hype, and Harm at the Dawn of Medicine's Computer Age* (New York: McGraw-Hill Education, 2015), 127–67. My account is based on Wachter's more thorough and detailed discussion. See also

Michael C. Brannigan, "Despite Medical Advances, Keen Attention still Required," *Albany Times Union*, September 26, 2019, https://www.timesunion.com/opinion/article/Despite-medical-advances-keen-attention-still-14471619.php.

11. This highlighted section retells and summarizes the case as it is described in more detail in Wachter, *The Digital Doctor: Hope, Hype, and Harm at the Dawn of Medicine's Computer Age*, 127–167.

12. Wachter, *The Digital Doctor*, 141.

13. Wachter, *The Digital Doctor*, 144.

14. Wachter, *The Digital Doctor*, 145.

15. Wachter, *The Digital Doctor*, 156.

16. J. I. Westbrook et al., "Association of Interruptions with an Increased Risk and Severity of Medication Administration Errors," *Archives of Internal Medicine* 170, no. 8 (April 26, 2010):683–690.

17. F. Sasangohar, B. Donmez, A.C. Easty, A. C, and P.L. Trbovich, "The Relationship between Interruption Content and Interrupted Task Severity in Intensive Care Nursing: An Observational Study," *International Journal of Nursing* Studies 52, no. 10 (October 2015): 1573–1581.

18. Nicholas Carr, *The Glass Cage: Automation and Us* (New York: W.W. Norton & Company, 2014), 67.

19. Carr, *The Glass Cage*, 69.

20. One of the foremost critics of the technological imperative is the Calvinist theologian and social theorist Jacques Ellul. See his early masterpiece, *The Technological Society*, trans. John Wilkinson (New York: Knopf, 1964).

21. Max Tegmark, *Life 3.0: Being Human in the Age of Artificial Intelligence* (New York: Vintage Books, 2017), 27–29.

22. Consider higher education and the drive toward online learning. This is especially the case during our COVID-19 pandemic. However, a major problem in disembodied learning is that we have equated genuine knowledge and understanding with the accumulation of facts and data disassociated from their all-important historic, social, cultural, philosophical, religious, economic, and political contexts. Rather than reflecting deeply on some issue, we learn in abbreviated, bullet-point fashion. It takes patience and the right aptitude to connect the dots and to ponder from various perspectives, particularly conflicting ones. This takes time, time that our standardized learning does not allow. Grades surely matter—to a degree. But a student's C, ever more rare with unremitting grade inflation, does not measure that student's capability and understanding. Nevertheless, the grade is what the test reveals. So also with patients.

23. Martha C. Nussbaum, *Frontiers of Justice. Disability, Nationality, Species Membership* (Cambridge, MA; London, UK: Belknap Press), 2006.

24. Michael C. Brannigan, *Cultural Fault Lines in Healthcare: Reflections on Cultural Competency* (Lanham, MD: Lexington Books, Rowman & Littlefield, 2012), 39–40; for a thoughtful critique of metrics in medicine, see Jerry Z. Muller, *The Tyranny of Metrics* (Princeton, NJ: Princeton University Press, 2018), 103–23.

25. Milan Kundera, *Slowness*, trans. Linda Asher (New York: HarperCollins, 1995), 2.

26. Kundera, *Slowness*, 2.

27. Kundera, *Slowness*, 39.

28. Jennifer Robertson, *Robo sapiens japanicus* (Oakland: University of California Press, 2018), 19; this was clearly the impetus behind former Prime Minister Shinzo Abe's *Innovation 25* policy, at Robertson, *Robo sapiens japanicus*, 29.

29. Darlei Dall'Agnol, "Caring Robots," blog for *Practical Ethics*, Oxford University, June 25, 2015; http://blog.practicalethics.ox.ac.uk/2015/06/guest-post-caring-robots.

30. Abraham Verghese, "Culture Shock—Patient as Icon, Icon as Patient," *New England Journal of Medicine* 359, no. 26 (Dec. 25, 2008): 2748–51.

31. Cassell, *Doctoring*, 71.

32. Cassell, *Doctoring*, 67.

33. Cassell, *Doctoring*, 67–68.

34. Rasha Al-Lamee, David Thompson, Hakim-Moulay Dehbi, Sayan Sen, Kare Tang, John Davies et al., "Percutaneous Coronary Intervention in Stable Angina (ORBITA): A Double-Blind Randomized Controlled Trial," *The Lancet* 391, no. 10115 (Jan. 6, 2018): 31–40, https://doi.org/10.1016/S0140-6736(17)32714-9.

35. Making eye contact and really listening are key to connect with the patient. And by eye contact, I do not mean staring. Staring directly into another's eyes is not only offsetting, but rude. Eye contact means looking at the patient.

36. Atsushi Senju and Mark H. Johnson, "Is Eye Contact the Key to the Social Brain?" *Behavioral and Brain Sciences* 33, no. 6 (2010): 458; cited in Sherry Turkle, *Reclaiming Conversation: The Power of Talk in a Digital Age* (New York: Penguin Press, 2015), 170.

37. Batya Friedman and Peter H. Kahn, Jr., "Human Agency and Responsible Computing: Implications for Computer System Design," *Journal of Systems and Software* 17, no. 1 (January 1992): 11.

38. Friedman and Kahn, "Human Agency and Responsible Computing," 11.

39. Ernest Becker, *The Denial of Death* (New York: The Free Press, 1973), 17.

40. Michael Ayrton, *The Maze Maker* (Chicago, IL: University of Chicago Press, 1967), 12.

41. Tegmark, *Life 3.0*, 29.

42. Blay Whitby, "Do You Want a Robot Lover? The Ethics of Caring Technologies," in *Robot Ethics: The Ethical and Social Implications of Robotics*, ed. Patrick Lin, Keith Abney, and George A. Bekey (Cambridge, MA: The MIT Press, 2012), 246; see also David Levy, *Love and Sex with Robots: The Evolution of Human-Robot Relations* (New York: HarperCollins, 2007).

43. Turkle, *Reclaiming Conversation*, 415. My remarks on the notion of "as-if" are influenced by Sherry Turkle's work and eye-opening insights. Turkle attributes the influence of Helene Deutsche, "Some forms of emotional disturbance and their relationship to schizophrenia," *Psychoanalytic Quarterly* 11 (1942): 301–21. Deutsche proposed the "as-if," or *als ob*, personality as one who essentially experiences a loss of "object cathexis," i.e., a loss of interest in the things and people in the world. She lays a foundational way of understanding what we call Borderline Personality Disorder. My use of the term "as if" is not in the context of this neurosis in its extreme expressions. It is more of the general, everyday delusions we convey

when we anthropomorphize objects such as robots and living beings such as pets, and, as such, has the potential to bring about some level of existential and interpersonal dysfunction.

44. Tegmark, *Life 3.0*, 86–89.

45. Tegmark, *Life 3.0*, 90–91.

46. For an interesting account of performance and Japanese robotics see Yuji Sone, *Japanese Robot Culture: Performance, Imagination, and Modernity* (New York: Palgrave, 2017).

47. Cited in Wallach and Allen, *Moral Machines*, 43.

48. Turkle, *Reclaiming Conversation*, 341.

49. Breazeal, *Designing Sociable Robots*.

50. Turkle, *Reclaiming Conversation*, 352.

51. Wallach and Allen, *Moral Machines*, 33–34.

52. Drew McDermott, "Why Ethics Is a High Hurdle for AI," paper at 2008 North American Conference on Computing and Philosophy, Bloomington, IN, July 12, 2008; cited in Wallach and Allen, *Moral Machines*, 35.

53. Wallach and Allen, *Moral Machines*, 26.

54. Carol Gilligan, *In a Different Voice: Psychological Theory and Women's Development* (Cambridge, MA: Harvard University Press, 1982).

55. Nel Noddings, *Caring: A Feminine Approach to Ethics and Moral Education* (Berkeley, CA: University of California Press, 1984).

56. American Nurses Association, "What Is Nursing?," accessed Feb. 6, 2020, https://www.nursingworld.org/practice-policy/workforce/what-is-nursing.

57. Mary Lou Peck, "The Future of Nursing in a Technological Age: Computers, Robots, and TLC," *Journal of Holistic Nursing* 10, no. 2 (June 1, 1992): 183.

58. See Rozzano C. Locsin and Hirokazu Ito, "Can Humanoid Nurse Robots Replace Human Nurses?" *Journal of Nursing* 5, no. 1 (2018), at http://www.hoajonline.com/nursing/2056-9157/5/1.

59. Roseangela Barcaro, Martina Mazzoleni, and Paolo Virgili, "Ethics of Care and Robot Caregivers," *Prolegomena* 17 (2018) 1: 76, doi:10.26362/20180204.

60. John Loeffler, "Should We Fear Artificial Intelligence?" *Interesting Engineering*, Feb. 23, 2019, https://interestingengineering.com/should-we-fear-artificial-superintelligence.

61. Loeffler, "Should We Fear Artificial Intelligence?"

62. Tony Prescott, "Me in the Machine," *New Scientist* 335, no. 3013 (March 2015): 36, https://doi.org/10.1016/S0262-4079(15)60554-1.

63. Prescott, "Me in the Machine," 38.

64. Aimee van Wynsberghe, "Designing Robots for Care: Care Centered Value-Sensitive Design," Science and Engineering Ethics 19 (2013): 427.

65. Pandora's container eventually endured as Pandora's "box" due to a later mistranslation of *pithos*, "jar," to *pyxis*, "box."

66. Isaac Asimov, "Runaround," in *Astounding Science Fiction*, March 1942: 94–103.

67. Isaac Asimov, *Robots and Empire* (Garden City, NY: Doubleday, 1985).

68. The late Joel Feinberg described these other types of harm in detail in the context of issues in medical ethics. See especially his masterful *Harm to Self*, Volume 3 in his *Moral Limits of the Criminal Law* (New York: Oxford University Press, 1986), and *Harmless Wrongdoing*, Volume 4 in *Moral Limits of the Criminal Law* (New York: Oxford University Press, 1990).

69. Robertson, *Robo sapiens japanicus*, 133.

70. National Society of Professional Engineers®, "Code of Ethics for Engineers," accessed Nov. 28, 2020, http://www.mtengineers.org/pd/NSPECodeofEthics.pdf.

71. Robert Sparrow and Linda Sparrow, "In the Hands of Machines? The Future of Aged Care," in *Minds and Machines* 16, no. 2 (2006): 141–61.

Chapter Four

What Is in a Face?

An unknown Athenian vase painter celebrated for his distinct red figures, dubbed the Niobid Painter (fl. 460–450 BCE), portrayed the creation of Pandora on one of his vases. As we recall, on the orders of Zeus, the artisan god Hephaestus created an artificial female, Pandora, out of earth and water, totally humanlike in appearance and behavior. On the upper panel of the vase, the painter depicts Pandora facing outward in full-frontal expression. This is a rarity in ancient Greek art. All other figures on the vase bear the typical side-view profile. In her exquisite book Gods and Robots, classical folklorist Adrienne Mayor tells us that faces shown sideways express life and energy. In contrast, full-frontal facial images convey what is inanimate, spiritless, static, without mind. Pandora's frontal gaze looks almost hypnotic. Her face appears to have either a slight smile or a leer, uncommon since faces in Greek art are usually expressionless.[1] Not so with Pandora.

Facial depiction in ancient Greek art is distinct from how we now think of the face. Our faces are the physical conduits for communicating. We carry out a face-to-face choreography in our shared dance. Philosopher Gabor Csepregi describes this cadence in his *The Clever Body*, "The face is a dialectical mimetic surface: it can translate both the content of, and the response to, a message."[2] Our world now also communicates through interactive digital technologies. Such technologies attempt to simulate this "mimetic quality," or dance. Consider the ubiquitous *emoji*, of which we send over five billion to each other daily. The Oxford English Dictionary christened *emoji*, meaning "picture character," 2015's Word of the Year. The word's Japanese origin highlights the culture's emphasis on non-verbal cues, particularly facial—facial muscles, eyes, cheeks, lips, and mouth. Our faces speak louder than words. The Japanese high-context language, deeply situational, underscores circumstance over words, context over content. The face reveals both inner and outer context. As Erving Goffman puts it, there are certain "traffic rules of interaction." The Japanese conversational style, deliberately indirect, involves facework in that how one shows his or her face is especially meaningful within a social context. There are therefore publicly acceptable parameters for showing one's feelings like joy, frustration, anger, or fear. Digital communication offers that safe place. Including emoji as a display of one's feelings is perfectly acceptable, just as singing a song out loud is encouraged in the proper setting of a karaoke bar, another Japanese invention.

Emoji also invites exchange. The emoji one sends, like any of those many renditions of the face, is reciprocated with another face or image, and the beat goes on. Emoji have become our own personal emotional translator. But not like the real, flesh-blood-and-bone face. As Csepregi astutely notes, the real face translates "both the content of, and the response to, a message." We learn the first steps of this unspoken art of translation early in infancy, a period when, as anthropologist Harvey Sarles asserts, the seeds of our morality are planted.

> the very basis of our moral being is located in the necessity of the m/other to have her developing child take on the moral equivalent of her responsibility for her infant. The child must begin to see itself as its m/other would: a sense of conscience, a sense of/for itself which sees itself.[3]

According to Sarles, through a dynamic interaction with the mother or surrogate the infant first attaches itself to and then separates from the mother, becoming a social self, which, for Sarles, takes on a moral fabric of conscience and responsibility for itself and others. Just as the mother gazes upon the face of her child, the infant gazes in return upon the face of the mother, especially her eyes and mouth. The child attends to the world through this interchange with the mother. This interaction shapes the child's individuality through a symbiotic interplay of gaze and gesture. Sarles: "M/other's glances, for example, effectively direct her child to look where she wants, then back at her. Much of this process is about sound, but also involves faces and eye directives and games . . . On our way to the emergence of the social-moral self, I suggest that the m/other utilizes the attachment process to direct her child to the world."[4] As the child develops its own sense of self through a gradual separating, developing its muscles and beginning to crawl around, sit upright, and walk, the child views itself as its own person, and, like mother, develops a sense of care and conscience as its world opens up to others.

Throughout our lives, face and body remain tangible cues that make all the difference in the quality of communication. At wakes and memorial services, words go only so far, as do cards and online condolences. Physically being there in person means more. Bodily cues have their own language. Our eyes, touch, embrace, physical demeanor, appearance, and silences convey a deeper meaning, cognitive and emotional, a nakedness stirring a near-immediate response, not altered over time as in interactive communication technologies like *emoji*. How we communicate in this Fourth Industrial Age of Big Data, artificial intelligence, and robotics is an existential gauge for how we see ourselves as humans and how we humans relate to our machines. Current and future interactive communication technologies raise a much higher bar than simple emoji. This is clearly the case with artificial intelligence and bold efforts to build what Max Tegmark calls "artificial general intelligence" (AGI), AI that replicates human intelligence, having "the ability to accomplish any cognitive task at least as well as humans."[5] For instance, as described earlier, *we each experience our illness in our own ways*. No person's experience is identical to another's. Will AI detect this subjectivity? Clues to our singular experience of illness are embodied, in the flesh. The body manifests not only what lies under the skin, but the immeasurable being who lives the illness. And the most telling bodily feature is that mystifying topography that unreflexively reveals our hidden climate—the face. Can AI read a human face, pick up on those subtle and not-so-subtle cues, like tone of voice, looks of apprehension, confusion, worry, fear? As we force-feed AI with prodigious mountains of data about medical history, genetics, and test results, the results are astounding and dazzlingly efficient. The power of super AI gives pause to human intelligence. We humans feed data into the machine, at least for now. But are we becoming redundant?

WELCOME TO THE UNCANNY VALLEY

This brings us to carebots, the prospect of their having humanlike faces, and the notion of the "uncanny valley." ReThink Robotics' collaborative "cobot" (co-worker robot) Baxter and its later sibling Sawyer set the pace with their screen faces and expressive eyes. The company shut down in 2018, but research continues. And after unveiling its humanoid robot Sophia in 2016, Hong Kong's Hanson Robotics developed the healthcare robot Grace in 2021. Grace with a face wears a nurse's uniform, has Asian features, and, the result of isolation during the pandemic, is targeted to interact with elders and others in confined settings.[6] Roboticists like Hiroshi Ishiguro are designing robots having real-looking human faces and hands. He and others are creating androids, robots more humanlike in appearance and behavior, artificial systems "designed with the ultimate goal of being indistinguishable from humans in its external appearance and behavior."[7] Ishiguro had earlier created his Geminoid (from the Latin *geminus*, "twin"), a matching copy of himself, a giant step forward in replicating specific individuals. He himself teleoperates Geminoid through attached devices. It is likely that carebots in the future will have human faces. If so, will sophisticated carebots with human faces better enable interaction between the robot caregiver and the human being cared-for?

When Japanese roboticist Masahiro Mori published his article, *Bukimi no Tani*, in 1970, it unleashed tidal waves of iterations and interpretations, especially among Western scholars. *Bukimi no Tani*, commonly translated as "uncanny valley," literally means "valley" (*tani*) of "eerie feeling," or "bad" (*bu*) "feeling" (*kimi*). "Uncanny" is not the best translation. Jennifer Robertson, conducting first-hand research in the field of human-robot interface, points out that Mori's *bukimi no tani* has no strong ties with Freud's notion of "uncanny," imbedded within the Austrian's psychoanalytic account of infantile repression to explain the sense of 'strange yet familiar,' *unheimlich*.[8] Also bear in mind that at the time of Mori's essay, 1970, typical bots were those industrial, clunky machines with little human likeness. Even now with the development of sophisticated humanoids, there are only a few places in Japan where human-robot interaction occurs, places like nursing homes, malls, hospitals, some hotels, and Tsukuba University's well-known robotics center and museum. At present, there is little in the way of real-life evidence to test Mori's *bukimi no tani*. Be assured, this will come.

In his essay, Mori uses a mountain-climbing analogy whereby unexpected terrain throws the climber into unknown territory. He claims that the more humanlike our machines become making them more familiar, this comfortable familiarity crosses a line when the similarity is so startling it generates a weird, unsettling feeling. Mori poses a simple graph with two vectors: human likeness (affinity) and comfort level. An increase in affinity brings about an increase in comfort. However, when affinity becomes too real, the comfort level dips downward, slipping into the "valley of eeriness." Similarity brings comfort, *up to a point*. Perfect humanlikess seems nonhuman. This is not at all like the initial response to identical twins, biologically natural clones, almost perfect copies. Their likeness compels us to actively seek some mark of distinction. My sisters are identical twins who have grown up and gelled together to become exceptionally first-class dancers.[9] The Brannigan twins' uncanny similarity runs deep. But nothing like a robot's uncanniness, machines from the start.

Appearance, Behavior, and Expectations

Not all humans will undergo discomfort. Much rests upon the user's subjectivity. Nonetheless, the face plays a climactic role. The more the robot's face becomes human, something nonhuman creeps in. Is this not the case in our ordinary interaction with each other when there may be something about the other's face that appears disturbing, perhaps menacing? What is it about certain people that generates in others a sense of threat and untrustworthiness?

What brings about a sense of creepiness? As with human-to-human interaction, much depends upon the appearance of the carebot as well as its behavior, both verbal and non-verbal. For instance, though not a carebot, Ishiguro's Geminoid has a striking facial resemblance to Ishiguro, but is essentially a remote-controlled marionette. Having appearance but not behavior, it lacks the capacity for agency. His doppelgänger has a physical presence, but its social presence is minimal. Experiments in communicating with Geminoid reveal "action at a distance." That is, it is merely "there," and the user is aware of its being-there, which is not by itself genuine presence.[10] It may look at me, but it does not *see* me. As the object of its look, I may feel solace, worry, or nothing at all. Yet this is not due to the Geminoid, but to myself, my subjectivity, my awareness of being looked at. The Geminoid has no real interest in me although it looks *as if* it does.

A robot's appearance and level of agency influence expectations. Though a carebot is incapable at this point of the moral agency of humans, its human face can generate in the human user an *expectation* of a thin layer of moral agency, a minimalist version that involves at least *appearing* to be morally sensitive. If the face is such that the carebot appears morally insensitive, this can be unsettling for the one who is cared-for given the deeply moral context of caring. Again, consider human-to-human interaction. Human caregivers can perfunctorily *perform* acts of caring, or caretaking—lifting, bathing, feeding, etc.—without seeming to genuinely care. In caring contexts, "mechanical" and "uncaring" are synonymous. Philosophers Jeremy Fischer and Rachel Fredericks insightfully describe mechanistic acting in the context of moral sensitivity.[11] Caregiving acts are ambiguous. When the person being cared-for senses this ambiguity in a human caregiver, unease, apprehension, eeriness, even alarm can creep in. These human-to-human encounters offer clues as to how *not* to design a robot, particularly a caring robot. Mori thereby cautions us: When it comes to robots that more closely replicate a human face and hands, be careful how far you go. He uses the example of shaking hands with someone who wears a myoelectric prosthetic hand that feels so real, so natural it initially feels unnerving when one shakes hands with it.[12] Indeed, there is something distinctive about the human hand. Martin Heidegger heeded this in his essay "What Is Called Thinking?" when he posed a natural association between thought and "handiwork" (*Handwerk*), an associative sort of bond between hands, tools, and mind. Mori's warning: our efforts to completely simulate ourselves can backfire.

With this vibrant synergy among appearance, behavior, and expectations, users' anticipations play a major role in the quality of the human-robot interaction. What do we look forward to from a caring companion? If designers of carebots intend to design a caring robot with a human face and human voice, we may naturally expect 'someone' approachable, responsive, and empathic.

"Someone" that sees me and recognizes me, not just looks at me. As for voice, we have been already primed to interact with a bot. Nicholas Carr comments on the eager acceptance and appeal of Alexa and its clever mythic connection with Amazon's Echo, "Every Narcissus deserves an Echo." Voice lies at the edge of any uncanny valley.[13] As we increasingly default to "speak with" Alexa and share with our chatbot, we humans are more easily bonding by way of the machine's voice. For those being cared-for, this need for recognition is crucial. Though recognition *per se* does not generate empathy, it offers a necessary bridge to empathy. As sociologist Stanley Cohen puts it, *acknowledging* the Other is a far cry from mere "knowledge" of the Other.[14] We will look more closely at empathy later on.

Anthropomorphism is unquestionably at play here. Our age-old, seemingly innate drive to attribute some humanness to nonhuman entities, even to what is beyond-human as we fashion our deities in our image, illustrates this synergy among appearance, attribution, and expectations. To a smiling face we attribute a pleasant disposition and expect a modicum of "friendliness." How a carebot looks will no doubt influence our assumptions, attributions, and expectations. And how a carebot functions is expected to be congruent with how it looks. What especially rings out is that a caring robot's non-personality disappears once it has a human face. A face erases anonymity. It also attests to the primacy of our perception in symbiotic interaction with the other. Any sense of weirdness we may feel creeps in when we perceive incongruence, imbalance, and disproportionality, something unexpected. Facial features can convey this sense of mismatch from what we expect. At the same time, in view of our innate anthropomorphic disposition toward nonliving objects and nonhuman living entities like pets, insects, etc., this is self-revealing. Well-measured studies like those of communication scholars Byron Reeves and Clifford Nass support this tendency we have of attributing human qualities to the nonhuman through what they call our "media equation." For instance, with computers we unthinkingly apply social codes of human conduct.[15] We complain kicking and screaming at our computer, "It's acting up again." At the mall, would you donate money to a charity if a robot asks you with a male or a female voice? The voice we choose for our GPS reveals our comfort level to more freely interact with it. Our choices, our personal biases, for better or worse, reveal our ground rules for interacting. In like manner, if those who are cared-for could choose the gender, face, ethnicity, and voice of their caring robot, they will most likely choose one with which they feel more comfortable. Otherwise, there is no ground for trust.

Proximity, Gaze, and Mind

As for the synergy among appearance, behavior, and expectations, replicating human appearance and behavior in ways that will better evoke a seamless interaction with users runs into some heavy challenges. University of Auckland's Elizabeth Broadbent describes two: proximity and gaze. These are obstacles between humans as well. In human-to-human interaction, we presume a certain social code, what we normally expect in proxemics (distancing), conversation, and interpersonal presence, admitting of cultural variables. When we violate such codes, we disrupt interactive equilibrium. Yet we expect a similar code with robots. The uncanny valley notion stresses that robots are not meant to be too much like us, underscoring the paradox that the more they resemble us, the more Other, alien, they may become. Resemblance too close for comfort sparks that "Promethean shame" philosopher Günther Anders describes we feel when encountering our "perfect" creation.[16]

First, the hurdle of proximity. We humans value our personal space in interacting with others. This is relationally and cultural toned. Certain cultures are closer in face proximity than others. Take the apparently simple act of approach. What is involved in the ways we approach each other is in fact enormously complex. In Maurice Merleau-Ponty's penetrating account of motility, movement is inherently intentional. Approaching some Other possesses its own momentum within a unified dynamic between mover and moved-to, approacher and approached. The approach is not driven by consciousness of approaching, but by the "momentum of existence."

> Sight and movement are specific ways of entering into relationship with objects and if, through all these experiences, some unique function finds its expression, it is the momentum of existence, which does not cancel out the radical diversity of contents, because it links them to each other, not by placing them all under the control of an "I think," but by guiding them towards the intersensory unity of a "world." Movement is not thought about movement, and bodily space is not space thought of or represented.[17]

Merleau-Ponty more explicitly maintains this notion of momentum when he emphasizes:

> Motility, then, is not, as it were, a handmaid of consciousness, transporting the body to that point in space of which we have formed a representation beforehand. In order that we may be able to move our body towards an object, the object must first exist for it, our body must not belong to the realm of the "in-itself."[18]

Engineering the approach of the nonhuman body of a caring robot toward an embodied human presents a major technical challenge, for the human body is not merely "*in* space, or *in* time. It *inhabits* space and time."[19]

The second hurdle Broadbent describes is that of seeing, or gaze behavior. The variety of gazes is unquenchably rich—the quick glance, the more prolonged look, the scan, etc. In Western cultures, we customarily expect eye-to-eye exchange in interacting with others. This combined with gesture, body language, and hand and arm movement are spontaneous body signals that say more than words. With a carebot, however, we are not quite sure what to expect, so that an eye-to-eye gaze can be disturbing. But avoiding eye contact can be just as disconcerting. Still, communication surpasses utterance and performance. Can a carebot replicate this communication sufficiently for the user to engage with the carebot? Will it be enough for the user to trust the carebot?[20] After all, the gaze suggests the potential for mentation. A robot with a human face evokes the possibility of mind because a living human face suggests mental activity, particularly via certain features and degrees of movement of eyes, etc. Its gaze signals to the perceiver a "gazer." Its uttering a response signals a "responder." (Unless the perceiver is an ardent Buddhist, in which case the assumption of some subject or thinker behind the act remains a misguided bias.) In other words, the face signifies a private portrait of agency, one that comprises mentation, experience, and response, that is, a mental life.[21] Notions of agency force us to re-think the question of "moral agency" and its myriad ethical concerns—privacy, harm, personhood, moral and legal culpability, responsibility, autonomy, etc. But these concerns pull us away from our present phenomenological, existential focus. The question lies not in whether and to what degree there is mental activity in the robot. This is daunting enough technically with ongoing efforts to stretch AI to simulate consciousness. Our principal phenomenological and existential concern lies in the degree to which humans, particularly those being cared-for, perceive a thinking carebot. Will the cared-for think that their caring robot thinks? It is the face that triggers this possibility of intelligence as the carebot sees and responds to the human user. The face represents an agentic capacity that a robot exhibits via communicating, memory, and recognition. Such performative features, though simulated, certainly manifest, as in the case of Paro and nursing home residents, degrees of 'mind,' or consciousness as subjective experience as Max Tegmark minimally describes it, that we attribute to the robot.[22]

An early study (2013), the first to investigate how facial differences on bots affected viewers' attribution of personality, found that human subjects assigned more personality and mind-like qualities to a robot with a human face. Subjects actually preferred interacting with this type of robot as long as the face conveyed a comfortable level of trustworthiness. The methodology was straightforward. Subjects interacted randomly with a wheel-operated and touch-screen Peoplebot healthcare robot under three conditions: 1) the screen displayed a human face, 2) the screen displayed a human silver face, and 3) the screen displayed no face at all, simply designated as a Healthcare robot.[23] Subjects clearly preferred condition 1. They least preferred condition 2, the silver face, perceiving it as the eeriest of the three. Humanlikeness in itself does not generate a sense of uncanny. What matters is the *kind* of human face. The silver face, while human in form, is incongruent, not what we expect. We naturally wonder: Is this human or not?

Here again is the technical challenge designers face in constructing a robot's face, especially a carebot. As the above study concludes,

> Designers need to think carefully about what qualities they wish their robot to be perceived as having and design the face accordingly. A humanlike face display should be used if the designers wish the robot to be perceived as having greater abilities to experience things, have agency and be seen as more sociable and amiable. On the other hand, if the designers do not want people to have high expectations of the robot having these abilities, then a humanlike face display may not be useful.[24]

What impressions on the part of the user are desired? As a sidebar, why presume that elders even want their caring robot to have a human face? Some do not. Residents in care institutions should therefore have a choice. Still, the kind of face matters. Broadbent and others have underscored that human affinity or likeness is not *per se* the determinative factor in feelings of oddness. Rather, it is the *perceived personality*, or mind-quality, that the face mirrors that can be off-putting. It disrupts the expectation of a warm, friendly, kind, empathic, and most importantly, trusting personality of a carebot. Like the kind of face that Josie immediately spots in Klara when the artificial friend looks out from the shop window in Ishiguro's *Klara and the Sun*. Though Ishiguro does not describe Klara's face, it is Klara's face that makes Josie want Klara as her friend, her real friend. So here is the phenomenological rub: When I look at the carebot's face, do I think of it as looking back at me? For Levinas, as we will see, *le visage*, while beyond the physical face *in toto*, is still grounded upon the embodied physical face that represents the irreducibility of the Other.

In short, can we capture a face that is *human enough* to be user-friendly, but, sliding away from literal realism, *not too human*. Otherwise, *bukimi* can seep in to become an obstacle in our interaction with robots. The challenge is daunting, not only because of the delicacies in human motility, but in tough snags when designing a face with its countless nuances. Take the human smile, abundantly intricate, so complex that it is at times difficult to distinguish a smile from a grimace or from a leer. Is Pandora's face a smile or a leer? A smile is not just a smile. Adriano Angelucci, Pierluigi Graziani, and Maria Grazia Rossi take us under the hood of a smile, noting the natural symphony of facial muscles, cartilage, blood flow, complexion, skin, and fat.

> Facial muscles are over 30, about a dozen of which are involved in smiling. The contraction of each of these muscles during a smile varies greatly in speed, intensity, and direction; it hinders or facilitates the contraction of nearby muscles, and propagates to facial cartilages. This complex pattern of forces is then transmitted to the skin . . . As a consequence of this complexity, skin behavior can easily become unmanageable. Compressing and stretching the skin alters the blood flow and gives rise to different skin complexions, thereby making blood vessels more or less visible. Depending on elasticity, collagen percentages, and other concurrent factors, including highly subjective ones such a habitual facial expression, wrinkles, and (possibly) scars may also become more or less visible. Stretched skin, on the other hand, tends to make facial bones more visible.[25]

And so on. You get the picture. A carebot's smile can be off-putting.

How can we invite a comfortable enough human-robot exchange that allows for the perception of carebot sensitivity and empathy? Angelucci and colleagues argue that the better model to study human-machine interaction is via computer simulation. Though not directly applicable to carebots, their claim is grounded upon how we interface with our devices. Whether robots or computers, our human-machine interface reveals more regarding us than about the machine. Indeed, interacting with robots offers a rich opportunity to better understand ourselves on cognitive and social levels. As they point out, "precisely *because* of the uncanny, androids may turn out to provide the best means of finding out what kinds of behaviors we perceive as human."[26] Moreover, they add that our own human reluctance to recognize an Other that appears in some disconcerting, non-human way impedes any possibility for empathic interaction, a foundational feature in genuine caring.

Familiarity induces comfort. Ontologically, no one else is *me*. There is an ever-present divide between you and me, what I call our "original fault line."[27] Nevertheless, as an evolutionary habit, we feel more at ease, more at home, with those *like us*, other humans. Undoubtedly this spawns a dark side—those not like us remain strangers. Yet the comfort that comes with familiarity is conditional. A major condition lies in not crossing that line when likeness becomes so real it is unreal. *Bukimi no tani* ultimately refers to not crossing that line where simulation looks *too real*, so human it is non-human. Unnatural enough to induce anxiety, discomfort, and unsettledness, it counters any possibility for a nurturing human-robot interaction. This logically pulls us into the tricky conceptual terrain of so-called naturalness. What is "natural"? "Unnatural"? While worthy of extended discussion, we will not here go spelunking into its rich and cavernous tomes of research, even though it pretty much drives our core question—What makes us human? Moreover, whether our initial shock at realizing the artificiality of an all-too-natural feeling hand remains disturbing enough to be a chink in the human-robot interface remains arguable. Indeed our human history is one of coming-to-terms. A coming-to-terms with new, offsetting, even blasphemous ideas. A coming-to-terms with the unanticipated, perhaps frightening, features of a partner's personality. A coming-to-terms with the otherness that is at first threatening. Mori's *bukimi no tani* pertains less to the machine or robot but more to the human who encounters it.

Uncanny Valley is, at its core, a metaphorical reference to our individual, unique, and acculturated subjectivity when interfacing with a machine. This interfacing is not between two completely separate entities, human and machine, but a dynamic relationality through which the human extends self-awareness outside the typically confined composite of the physical, body-schema morphology, similar to Andy Clark's thesis of "extended mind." In his Foreword to Clark's *Supersizing the Mind*, David Chalmers cites his iPhone to illustrate how an object "is not my tool, or at least it is not wholly my tool. Parts of it have become parts of me."[28] In their original article introducing their "extended mind" thesis, they describe it in terms of "active externalism."

> In these cases, the human organism is linked with an external entity in a two-way interaction, creating a *coupled system* that can be seen as a cognitive system in its own right. All the components in the system play an active causal role, and they jointly govern behavior in the same sort of way that cognition usually does. If we remove the external component the system's behavioral competence will drop, just as it would if we removed parts of its brain. Our thesis is that this sort of coupled process counts equally well as a cognitive process, whether or not it is wholly in the head.[29]

Accompanying this self-extension (my wife Brooke prefers to call it "self-expression") is our innately variable human subjectivity, the fact that we each perceive in different, unique, nuanced, and subtle ways. We each inhabit our own bodiliness, and this naturally impacts *what* and *how* we see. This is why my experience of my illness, grounded upon my sense of incapacity, is strictly my own. Hence, the perennial challenge caregivers face, whether human or machine—that of somehow breaking through and entering through those banal cracks in the daily discourse of that 'other country' of the cared-for. In the same way, each of us will respond in our distinct ways to a carebot with human features, hands, face, and eyes. Each of us lives out a subjectivity carved out by our histories, our unfolding re-seeing and reinterpreting of selected memories, our imaginative sensibilities, our personhood of bodily and mental muscle, along with assimilated cultural imprints, bundles of ideas, beliefs, values, and heresies we have carried along the way. Jennifer Robertson is on point when she writes,

> It is reasonable to posit that not everyone reacts to a given thing in the same way—some may fall into a valley of their creation, others may not conjure such a valley at all. Mori treats the *bukimi no tani* response as a human universal, as if all humans were hardwired in the same way. It is more likely that other factors—such as physical and cognitive abilities, age, sex, gender, sexuality, ethnicity, education, religion, and cultural background—influence the way in which people respond to an unfamiliar sight or an extraordinary impression.[30]

Gesture, the Indispensability of Face, and Empathy

The approach is gesture, an exercise in motility. Gestures come in many guises: verbal, facial, body, etc. Gestures manifest our own personal language and bear witness to who we are as living creatures. Ludwig Wittgenstein, digging into the dynamic of words, understanding, and language, and recognizing the expressive power of gesture writes, "How curious: we should like to explain our understanding of a gesture by means of a translation into words, and the understanding of words by translating them into a gesture."[31] This natural interplay of speaking and gesturing sends a message: expression is, at its core, bodily. I see this in action whenever I return to Japan. Colleagues, friends, and family will not only affirm an observation with the conventional "*Hai*," or "*Hai. So desu.*" They will naturally express it with a slight forward nod of the head to whom they speak. They will even do this speaking on the phone. In Mediterranean cultures like Italy, this natural chemistry between speech and gesture is particularly evident. Gesture is a ballet with its stops and turns that embellishes what we say. Communicating involves both what and how we express it. Gesture is the how, a mimetic bodily clarifying that complements and rescues our speech. Simulating this dance of gesture is another monumental hurdle in designing carebots. Especially since caring is the litmus test of being human to each other in caring-for, caring-about, and giving care, ultimate and intimate communicative acts we do with our whole selves—spirit, will, heart, and body. Our bodies' inherent expressiveness conveys this universal truth: We all carry out our own choreography in our face-to-face waltz. We lead and are led, give and take, take turns improvising and sustaining the dance through our bodies, hands, and, most notably, our face.

How valuable is this embodied face-to-face interaction in a world of digital computer-mediated-communication? As the world came under the grip of COVID-19, digital forms of communication have become providential. Connecting with each other through our devices and screens was a blessing. But has it improved our quality of living? In an earlier 2011 study, communication scholars from three Chinese Universities (Hong Kong, Tsinghau, and Hauzhong) collected survey data from four cities—Hong Kong, Taipei, Beijing, and Wuhan—to compare two styles of communication, computer-mediated and face-to-face, in order to assess impact on quality of life. Residents in these four cities used the Internet quite extensively. Researchers aimed to ascertain "whether Internet communication can replace face-to-face interaction in enhancing quality of life."[32] They measured "quality of life" in terms of social support, leisure, life satisfaction, and interpersonal engagement. They initially hypothesized that information communication technologies (ICT) would most likely enhance quality of communication among users. Their findings revealed the opposite. Face-to-face communication was a more reliable predictor of quality of life among users than ICT. Face-to-face communication resulted in a much higher quality of life than communication through the Internet.[33] They discovered that what mattered was not the quantity of time one spends on either mode of communication, but the nature of the communication. As the authors state, citing the pivotal work of Ray Birdwhistle who, in pioneering the field of kinesics, the study of body-motion, emphasized the importance of non-verbal cues:

> The Internet cannot convey the 'warmth' of face-to-face communication ... the absence of non-verbal cues, lack of warmth, and less demand for engagement in Internet communication, which results in impersonality, shallow interactions, and difficulty in building social support, are reasons for the negative contribution of online communication to perceived quality of life.[34]

ICT is clearly more efficient. It also enables deliberate editing of how we present ourselves.

Yet even though face-to-face communication takes more effort and, due to its spontaneity one must deal with the unexpected, face-to-face communication offered a higher quality of life among participants. At heart, what counts are those non-verbal cues, gestures, body language, facial expressions, signals, or "tells" as in poker. The face, like a lighthouse beam, reveals, if the perceiver sees, one's inner state.

Without doubt, the benefits of having a carebot are considerable. But think carefully. What does it mean when the user talks *with*, not *to*, the bot? Is there a real conversation? Does the bot genuinely *understand* what we say? Caregiving entails a reflective capacity for empathy. Can a carebot offer empathy, the kind that comes with that face-to-face interaction with its multidimensional cues and nuances? Excavating the meaning of empathy is a challenge. It has become our fashionable term with all sorts of meanings depending upon the situation and described in distinct ways in fields as diverse as neuroscience, primatology, politics, and ethics. For instance, the clichéd "I feel your pain" is all-too-simplistic. Given its long history of interpretation, empathy wears many faces. Its origins stem from its 1890s formulation in German psychologist Theodore Lipps' *Einfühlung*, a type of "in-feeling" when facing an art form or object.[35] After various iterations, empathy has come to mean a kind of emotive resonance with another's experience. As a sort of understanding, sense, intuition or knowing to some extent what another feels, empathy means somehow situating ourselves inside the other.

How does this come about? The idea of a powerful connection between empathy and seeing is supported by neuroscientists who claim that empathy has to do with brain mechanisms, so-called mirror neurons, that activate in varying degrees when we witness another's act or when we ourselves perform that same act. In his *Mirroring People*, Italian neurologist Marco Iacoboni uses the example of seeing the infamous head-butting by France's Zinédine Zidane against an Italian opponent that led to Zidane's ejection from the 2006 World Cup final match and Italy's subsequent stunning victory over France. Iacoboni states that the billions of viewers who saw this palpably "felt" the hit and were drawn deeper into the match and outcome.[36] Due to this neuronal mirroring, we naturally situate ourselves within what we perceive. This is particularly the case when we see a face that looks happy, anxious, etc. Much depends upon the facial muscles, cheeks when smiling, brows when worried. In face-to-face interaction, we naturally activate our mirror neurons.

What if a person is facially paralyzed? Moebius syndrome is a rare congenital disorder that affects facial muscles. Though termed congenital facial diplegia, it is not typically inherited. Deficient and underdeveloped sixth and seventh cranial nerves inhibit normal facial expression and eye movement. There is no cure. Still, certain treatments enable those who have this condition to live on. Due to the variety of symptoms—trouble swallowing, cleft palate, hearing and dental problems, crossed eyes, etc.—lifelong treatment involves neurologists, otolaryngologists, ophthalmologists, plastic surgeons, and others. Basically, the condition brings about near complete paralysis of facial muscles. This means that the person cannot display facial expression like smiling, frowning, surprise, fear, etc.

What if a person chooses temporary facial paralysis? Consider a willfully chosen treatment that freezes facial muscles. Botox is a multibillion dollar industry. It enables us to diminish facial signs of aging. If we cannot stay young, at least we can avoid appearing old. The pressure on women is especially titanic given how much emphasis we place upon youth and beauty.

In our youth-productivity-oriented culture, aging brings with it a simple yet deadly equation: with aging comes, in this order, irrelevance, obsolescence, and invisibility. You can usually tell if someone has been "botoxed": a typically shiny, smooth, uncreased forehead. No lines, no wrinkles. To some the face may appear to carry a certain flatness. Because of the skin's tightness, the needled face loses much of its elasticity along with those micro-expressions that convey one's inner state—happiness, anger, sadness, fear, disgust, surprise. Facial muscles are essentially frozen in time. The face finds it difficult to unconsciously mimic others' facial expressions. If I undergo Botox treatment and you wince with pain, because my stiffened face cannot mimic yours, it is difficult for me to "feel your pain," and worse, *to show you that I feel it*, even if slightly. Though we can never literally feel another's pain, at least having some sense of another's pain, anger, happiness, or fear is a condition for empathy. And according to the mirror neuron theory, this mimicking begins early on. Imagine a botoxed mother interacting with her infant. What face does the infant see? A frozen, unresponsive face, restricts the child's way of engaging with the mother and eventually with the world.[37]

Our interior state is like a room, and in that room is a window out of which we look—the face. We generally manifest six basic windows when we express happiness, anger, fear, sadness, surprise, disgust and their various renditions. Our faces convey even the subtlest of hints. Others can peer into our room by looking through our window, our face. At best, the smiling emoji face offers a slight tap on the window. So how do mirror neurons enter in? Basically, when I see you smile, mirror neurons in my brain immediately fire so that I inwardly feel your smile along with you, a pre-reflective inner imitation. Mirror neurons instantly send signals to areas in my limbic area that controls emotion. These signals in turn enable me to smile. This inner simulation—feeling your smile and reacting—offer a possible neurological basis for empathy, feeling along with another, philosopher Kendall Walton's "other-shoe" imagining as if we were the other.[38] What is especially important is that I first *feel* the emotion that your smile conveys, and only later recognize the emotion. *Feeling comes first. Not cognition.* I do not first *know* you are happy and then feel happy with you. This is critically important in the matter of caring robots, algorithmically encoded to respond in specific ways within a fundamentally cognitive framework. We humans essentially feel first, and then reflect and respond. What happens neurologically is amazingly complex, an incredible cascade of neuronal activity that Iacoboni breaks down into movements along major brain areas. After mirror neurons simulate what we see, the insula acts as the pathway for these mirror neurons to connect with the limbic system. The amygdala in the limbic system is particularly receptive in the case of faces. Iacoboni sums up his hypothesis for this neuronal basis of empathy: "According to this mirror neuron hypothesis of empathy, our mirror neurons fire when we see others expressing their emotions, as if we were making those facial expressions ourselves. By means of this firing, the neurons also send signals to emotional brain centers in the limbic system to make us feel what other people feel."[39] That is pretty straightforward, even though the journey from mirror neurons to how we ourselves feel is exceedingly complex. Again, feeling precedes thought.

Despite empathy's many faces, Irish author Colum McCann captures it nicely when he writes, "The only true way to expand your world is to inhabit an otherness beyond ourselves. There is one simple word for this: *empathy*."[40] Empathy only comes about when we free ourselves from our private and protective world of "I, me, and mine." We humans can unshackle ourselves from our bubbles of self. Can robots? Can carebots break out of their algorithms? Do they even have a "world" to "expand"? A robot may respond *as if* it understands and feels along with the cared-for. The person cared-for, in turn, may respond *as if* there is a real conversation taking place without pretense. Nonetheless, as Sherry Turkle persists wisely in cautioning us, though we humans increasingly immerse ourselves in this "as-if" reality, particularly because this "as-if" reality seems safer than the real human world, is it?[41]

LE VISAGE

The face has a unique essence that lies beyond artificial representation. This is the primal, skeletal challenge robotics engineers face in replicating a human face. More than its physical symphony of nerves, muscle, tissue, and cartilage, the face possesses its own *élan vital*, its inner core in the spirit of Henri Bergson's vital impulse. Lithuanian-Jewish philosopher Emmanuel Levinas, in his metaphysics of ethics, insists on the transcendent quality of the face, *le Visage*. On one level, the human face is that all-too-common connective social tissue throughout the everyday course of human interaction. We see each other, and we relate to each other via our faces. On another level, our routine engagement reaches beyond ordinariness. The Other's face offers us the opportunity to peek through a crack in the discourse of the routine, pulling us beyond sameness. This moment constitutes a "rupture of being."[42]

Levinas' insight is remarkable from someone who survived a bitter ordeal in a prisoner-of-war camp, merely one among others in a brutally prevailing condition of "the Same," *la Même*. Even after Levinas' captivity at Fallingbostel, *la Même* cast its shadow when his family and that of his wife were snuffed out along with over one million others at Auschwitz. Nonetheless, though this has lingered on as his "tumor in the memory" in which Auschwitz and all its iterations—Bergen-Belsen, Dachau, etc.—mirrored unspeakable evil, he holds fast to an optimistic hope urging us to awaken to our innate capacity to see beyond and break free from the Same, to recognize the other's singularity and transcendence, the other's "beyond."

Caring for another involves being-with and being-for the other. Consider those caregiving interactions involving physical contact—lifting, turning the person in bed, bathing, cleaning, showering, feeding, etc. These are not merely physical, mechanical acts. They involve the intimacy of touch. Touch has its own healing power. These caregiving acts also involve seeing the one cared-for. Seeing is more than merely looking at the person. Seeing the other's face demands more than skimming the surface. It goes beyond a glance or brushed look. Seeing another's face, even camp guards, fractures the comfort of *la Même* in which all are faceless. Levinas cries out on behalf of all, particularly the marginalized, sentenced to facelessness in a narrative that levels the Other. Levinas reminds us that seeing another, particularly the other's face, pulls us into the other's flesh, blood, bone, and spirit, the other's aliveness. Levinas echoes Merleau-Ponty's persuasion that "It is the simple fact that I live in the facial expressions of the other, as I feel him living in mine."[43] Moreover, Levinas goes beyond the conviction. This encounter with the other's face is the "rupture of being," a liberation from the routine, from the oppressive world of sameness in which we tend to view the other as just like any other.

Behold Levinas' marvelous turn in which the face of the Other, in our case the person cared-for, testifies to a "beyond." Levinas describes an interhuman engagement in which a person recognizes, truly sees, the other. For a carebot to recognize this "beyond," it must free itself (the agency question) from the world of sameness so that its caregiving acts are not merely performances. Is this "rupture of being" even germane when it comes to artificial life, to the carebot? Among humans, this rupture shatters our customary way of seeing, one that reifies what is looked at, making the object of our look a static thing. In reality that "thing" is in essence dynamic, a living person, the person cared-for. Rupture of being = rupture in seeing. Seeing the face of the other reconfigures how we relate to the other.[44] This "rupture of being" constitutes the cornerstone in Levinas' metaphysics of ethics. For him, the face discloses a vulnerability and powerlessness that silently pleads to the seer "Do not harm," "Do not bring about unnecessary suffering." Though Levinas' concern is with all humans and does not single out elders, those being cared-for are particularly vulnerable. The encounter with the other's face remains an ever-present moral invitation. In his *Otherwise Than Being*, our moral accountability is fundamentally "asymmetric." That is, the encounter with the other's face is an embodied reminder of the moral responsibility we bear to the other. The other, likewise, bears the same to me. However, accountability must start somewhere. One of us must take the first step in this mutual moral obligation.

Our encounter with the face of the Other is, for Levinas, an epiphany, an awakening to my moral obligation. When it comes to caregiving, this obligation rests squarely upon the caregiver. The caregiver must take the first step. In this epiphany, faces of the cared-for and the caregiver, or any other face, leaves what Levinas terms a "trace," which is "not just one more word; it is the proximity of God in the countenance of my fellow man."[45] In his brilliant account of Levinas, journalist Salomon Malka powerfully articulates this "trace":

> It is divine commandment without divine authority . . . There is no uglier truth perhaps, but it needs to be said. *Levinas's phenomenology of the face of the Other in its ethical height receives its philosophical clarity in and from Fallingbostel, Bergen-Belsen and Auschwitz.* In the concentration camp, the "trace" of the face that, could it signify anything, would signify the divine commandment "Thou shalt not kill," becomes transparent in the clarity that only happens in an overcast afternoon.[46]

The face of the Other, in our case that of the cared-for, is the embodied conduit of this moral command which is all-inclusive, not exclusive to certain age cohorts, gender, race, cultures, ethnicities, religions, beliefs, citizenship, and other borders of superficial similitude or sameness.

Paradox: The Face Reveals and Conceals

This moral invitation braces Levinas' view that *le Visage* manifests a "transcendence" whereby the Other, as infinite, lies beyond our limited human encapsulation, outside of any philosophical system, ideology, or medical metrics. The face of the patient and the one cared-for is not just a physical face. It reflects an infinity, a mystery, neither seized nor quantified through data and tests. The Other's face is a canvas of the immeasurable. Truly seeing the Other's face awakens the seer to a transcendence that reveals concealment. The cared-for's face manifests the cared-for's mystery as person, whose reality lies beyond any algorithm, human or AI. Thus, the implicit paradox in the encounter. The face of the Other is there in flesh and bone, self-evident. And its embodied presence being-there is a concrete self-disclosure, a tangible truth. At the same time, the face of the Other conveys something hidden and unreachable. The cared-for's face both reveals and conceals.

Caregivers thereby face an obstinate challenge—truly seeing the cared-for, truly seeing the person's face. To genuinely see, one must yank oneself out of routine, reified, static, and metric molding. We need to see our elders' pain etched on their faces. We must recognize their anxiety and fear of being alone. Carebots also face the challenge, though unmindful of it. Can they be so designed to see the person they are caring for? To recognize the person's ineradicable beyond, transcendence, and mystery? By the same token, mutual co-presence calls for a presence to, for, and with each other. Can the user, the one cared-for, genuinely see the caregiver? The caregiver's concern, worry, frustration, relief, delight, empathy, compassion? Human caregivers have their "lines of pain," as we all. These, along with our lines of joy, are episodes from our unfolding private profiles. Seeing these lines further humanizes the caregiving experience and helps soothe the cared-for's pain. In Richard Selzer's "Parable," the dying patient sees a deep furrow across his doctor's forehead. Stunned to see that his doctor also suffers, he impulsively reaches up, touches his doctor's brow and strokes his doctor's "line of pain," "a look of wonder upon his face, as though he were just waking from a deep sleep."[47] With a caring robot, is any of this even possible? There are no lines of pain for a machine without a personal history. Yet the simulation may be good enough for the user. The person cared-for may believe in the carebot enough to tolerate the pretense.

My dear friend Hiroko Suzuki lives in Tono, a mountain village in the region of Tohoku, Japan. Tohoku's entire coastal region Shinriku and beyond was completely shattered from its devastating March 11, 2011 triple tragedy of earthquake, tsunami, and nuclear meltdown. When I worked there as a volunteer to help in the aftermath, Hiroko shared with me the plight of her mother and townspeople in nearby Sendai. She spoke in her quiet manner. As she poured me a cup of sake, her face told it all. It revealed her deep sadness, yet it also concealed her mystery. Matters of the heart and soul lie beyond understanding. In seeing Hiroko's face, I underwent an epiphany, a moral invitation to acknowledge her 'beyond' that was right there, at that moment, a moment that can never return, *ichigo ichie*. Levinas puts it straightforward.

> The epiphany of the other involves a signifyingness of its own independent of this meaning received from the world. The other comes to us not only out of the context, but also without mediation; he signifies by himself . . . This presence consists in coming towards us, in *making an entry* . . . the *phenomenon* by which the apparition of the other is also a face . . . the epiphany of a face is a *visitation*.[48]

Levinas' message enriches the meaning of caregiving. Genuinely seeing the other's face sparks awareness of the divine transparency in the encounter. In our caregiving, the face of the person who is cared-for is both seen and a window to what is unseen. Such is the pulsing paradox of the face. Its visibility permits access to what lies behind the face, the untold mystery of the Other, of Hiroko, of our elders and their history engraved on their faces. The face of the Other denotes physical presence and transcendence. It unveils the person who surpasses measurement.

> It is the sparkling jewel of the patient's embodied presence and our mutual co-presence to, for, and with each other. It is the gem of paradox. Our presence to, for, and with each other—embodied and emboldened through our faces—reveals the seen and the unseen, the spoken and the unspoken, what is embraced and what is untouchable. Our co-presence discloses the extraordinary in and through the ordinary, a "divine" in the gathering. Hence, the encounter as covenant.[49]

As Martin Buber maintains, our encounter with the Thou in the Other punctures our bubble of safety and frees us from ourselves. The human face is living proof of the Other's radical uniqueness, her singularity, her transcendence of the Same.

Throughout this discussion of uncanny valley, face, and our human-robot interaction, is my inquiry into what makes us human as distinct from robots tainted by an epistemological, ontic, and linguistic dualism? Is this an exercise in question-begging? In presuming an ontological distinction between human and robot, am I not just as culpable as the teens in Ishiguro's *Klara and the Sun* who, at the Interaction meeting, view and treat Josie's artificial friend Klara as a mere object, echoing David Levy's caution in his *Love and Sex with Robots* that how we treat out robots mirrors how we treat humans? Masahiro Mori may have been awry of this entrapment in a cognitive prison. It is important to note that Mori is an ardent student of Buddhism, specifically the Mahayana School and its extreme expression in Zen Buddhism. To what extent this has influenced his view of robotics is yet to be determined. Some scholars see a pronounced impact, and the relationship among Shinto, Japanese animism, Buddhism, and robotics is understudied and offers a rich field for research, one that Jennifer Robertson has begun to perceptively undertake. The enduring Buddhist vision of liberating the mind from its dualistic cage finds expression in Mori's idea of "mind-release" as applied to robotics. Tsukuba University's Takeshi Kimura claims that this view toward robotics in Mori's work compels us to re-think the human-robot interface as not a relation between two distinct separate entities, human—robot, especially since Buddhist teachings do not support the notion of some independent, separate "I" or self. (Clark's extended mind thesis is also pertinent.) Kimura rightfully points out Mori's emphasis on a necessary "backward step" of looking *inward* rather than outward for insight. Perception, that 'still point' of our inner state, reminds us of the perennial Buddhist warning in the *Dhammapada* that our minds are like elephants that can either be tamed or run wild. Kimura reminds us of the great Zen teacher Dogen's ultimate instruction: "To learn oneself is to forget oneself."⁵⁰ This helps explain Mori's caution against slipping into the "eerie valley" that comes from our excessive desire to recreate ourselves. As the classic motif in our ancient myths, the desire for perfection crosses a fateful line, and human hubris brings about its undoing.

What face will a caring robot have? We are, for better *and* worse, lured to our own kind, even if it is fake. We can tolerate the pretense. This interactive lure becomes more complex when carebots are designed to ask questions of the one who is cared-for. "Did you take your medication?" "Is there anything I can do for you?" "Do you need help getting out of bed?" "Can I bring you your dinner?" Performance takes on a darker shade inviting interpersonal engagement, particularly in our culture's ageist and xenophobic context that institutionalizes and segregates those Others. What is more, the user's familial context carves out a healthy or unhealthy gestalt. When children and good friends do not visit as often—grandpa is fine since his carebot will look after him—that distancing leads grandpa to interface further with the robot. When one is lonely, if a human is not there, the Other will do, perhaps even better. Caring robots, "someone" that simply "listens," offer an as-if presence, programmed so that we "connect" with them.⁵¹ We too are being programmed. The robot's human face, in contrast to *le visage's* moral invitation, beckons us and the person being cared-for to have a relationship with it *as if* it is a real human. When a robot or any device "presents itself as having a mind of its own," the rules of the game change.

NOTES

1. Adrienne Mayor, *Gods and Robots: Myths, Machines, and Ancient Dreams of Technology* (Princeton, NJ: Princeton University Press, 2018), 166.

2. Gabor Csepregi, *The Clever Body* (Calgary, Alberta, Canada: University of Calgary Press, 2006), 77.

3. Harvey Sarles, "The Genesis of Morality," *Religious Humanism* 41, no. 1 (September 2010): 43, http://huumanists.org/sites/huumanists.org/files/articles/Genesis%20of%20Morality%20-%20Sarles_0.pdf.

4. Sarles, "The Genesis of Morality," 6.

5. Max Tegmark, *Life 3.0: Being Human in the Age of Artificial Intelligence* (New York: Vintage Books, Penguin Random House LLC, 2017), 39.

6. Farah Master, "Meet Grace, the Healthcare Robot COVID-19 Created," *Reuters*, June 9, 2021, https://www.reuters.com/business/healthcare-pharmaceuticals/meet-grace-healthcare-robot-covid-19-created-2021-06-09/.

7. Karl F. MacDorman and Hiroshi Ishiguro, "The Uncanny Advantage of Using Androids in Cognitive and Social Science Research," *Interaction Studies* 7, no. 3 (2006): 298–99, http://www.macdorman.com/kfm/writings/pubs/MacDorman2006AndroidScience.pdf.

8. Jennifer Robertson, *Robo sapiens japanicus: Robots, Gender, Family, and the Japanese Nation* (Oakland, CA: University of California Press, 2018), 156.

9. Jack Wax, "Choreographed Lives: Twins Marie Robertson and Maggie Dethrow Share Their Love of Dancing, *Inside Columbia*, May 27, 2020, https://insidecolumbia.net/2019/11/21/choreographed-lives.

10. Paul Dumouchel and Luisa Damiano, *Living with Robots*, trans. Malcolm DeBevoise (Cambridge, MA: Harvard University Press, 2017), 149–150.

11. Jeremy Fischer and Rachel Fredericks, "The Creeps as Moral Emotion," *Ergo* 7, no. 6 (2020), 27 pages, available at SSRN: https://ssrn.com/abstract=3739193.

12. Mori's description of prosthetics demonstrates what was then and now a societal bias against disabled persons in Japan. Jennifer Robertson rightly stresses this in her account, *Robo sapiens japanicus*, 155.

13. Nicholas Carr, "These Are Not the Robots We Were Promised," *New York Times*, Sept. 9, 2017, https://www.nytimes.com/2017/09/09/opinion/sunday/household-robots-alexa-homepod.html.

14. Stanley Cohen, *States of Denial: Knowing about Atrocities and Suffering* (Cambridge, UK: Polity Press, 2001), 249–277.

15. Bryon Reeves and Clifford Nass, *The Media Equation: How People Treat Computers, Television, and New Media Like Real People and Places* (Stanford, CA: Center for the Study of Language and Information, Stanford University, 2003).

16. Günther Anders, *L'obsolescence de l'homme: Sur l'âme à l'époque de la deuxième revolution industrielle*, trans. Christophe David (Paris: Ivrea, 2001), 37; cited in Dumouchel and Damiano, 30.

17. Maurice Merleau-Ponty, *Phenomenology of Perception,* trans. Colin Smith (London: Routledge & Kegan Paul, 1962), 137.

18. Merleau-Ponty, *Phenomenology of Perception*, 139.

19. Merleau-Ponty, *Phenomenology of Perception*, 139.

20. The pioneering work of Paul Ekman remains pivotal in studies detecting deception through faces. See his *Emotions Revealed: Recognizing Faces and Feelings to Improve Communication and Emotional Life*, 2nd ed. (New York: Henry Holt and Company, Owl Books, 2003).

21. Whether mental activity is identical to brain activity, one of the theories to explain mind-brain relationship, remains in dispute, beyond the scope of this study. The mind-brain identity theory supports AI efforts to replicate mind.

22. Tegmark, *Life 3.0*, 314.

23. Elizabeth Broadbent et al., "Robots with Display Screens: A Robot with a More Humanlike Face Display Is Perceived to Have More Mind and Better Personality," *Plos One* 8, no. 8 (August 28, 2013): 3ff., https://doi.org/10.1371/journal.pone.0072589.

24. Broadbent et al., "Attitudes towards Health-Care Robots in a Retirement Village," *Australasia Journal of Aging* 31, no. 2 (June 2021): 115–20.

25. Adriano Angelucci, Pierluigi Graziani and Maria Grazia Rossi, "The Uncanny Valley: A Working Hypothesis," in *Social Robots: Boundaries, Potential, Challenges*, ed. Marco Nørskov(Surrey, UK: Ashgate Publishing Limited, 2016), 128.

26. Angelucci et al., 127. The article indicates that Maria Rossi is the original author of some of the ideas.

27. Michael C. Brannigan, *Cultural Fault Lines in Healthcare: Reflections on Cultural Competency* (Lanham, MD: Lexington Books, Rowman Rowman & Littlefield Publishing Group, Inc. 2016), 16.

28. Andy Clark, *Supersizing the Mind: Embodiment, Action, and Cognitive Extension* (Oxford: Oxford University Press, 2011), x.

29. Andy Clark and David Chalmers, "Appendix: The Extended Mind," in Clark, *Supersizing*, 222.

30. Jennifer Robertson, *Robo sapiens japanicus*, 159.

31. Ludwig Wittgenstein, *Zettel*, trans. G.E.M. Anscombe (Berkeley: University of California Press, 1970), 41e.

32. Paul S. N. Lee et al., "Internet Communication versus Face-to-face Interaction in Quality of Life Social Indicators Research," *Social Indicators Research* 100, no. 3 (February 2011): 375–89, doi 10.1007/s11205-010-9618-3.

33. Lee and his team examined possible reasons, one being that those who are already somewhat socially isolated tend to gravitate towards Internet communication. This goes back to whether primary responsibility lies with either the user or the product. However, instead, they found that "people who enjoy social interactions and social support offline are more likely to use the Internet for interpersonal communication." Lee, "Internet Communication Versus Face-to-face Interaction," 385.

34. Lee, "Internet Communication versus Face-to-Face Interaction," 385–86, 387.

35. Susan Lanzoni, *Empathy: A History* (New Haven, CT: Yale University Press, 2018), 9. Lanzoni offers an excellent account of the various meanings given to empathy.

36. Marco Iacoboni, *Mirroring People: The Science of Empathy and How We Connect with Others* (New York: Picador, Farrar, Straus and Giroux, 2008), 106–108.

37. Jessie Cole, "Botox Silences Women's Faces—and Freezes Out Empathy in Body Language," *The Guardian*, May 22, 2013, https://www.theguardian.com/commentisfree/2013/may/22/botox-silences-womens-faces-empathy.

38. Kendall L. Walton, *In Other Shoes: Music, Metaphor, Empathy, Existence* (Oxford: Oxford University Press, 2015), 3.

39. Iacoboni, *Mirroring People*, 119.

40. Colum McCann, *Letters to a Young Writer* (New York: Random House, 2017), 12.

41. Michael C. Brannigan, "On Robots, Depression, and the Lure of the Not-Quite-Real," *Times Union*, April 1, 2021.

42. Emmanuel Levinas, *Ethics and Infinity: Conversations with Philippe Nemo*, trans. Richard A. Cohen (Pittsburgh, PA: Duquesne University Press, 1985), 87.

43. Maurice Merleau-Ponty, "The Child's Relations with Others," in *The Primacy of Perception and Other Essays on Phenomenological Psychology, the Philosophy of Art, History and Politics*, trans. William Cobb, ed. James M. Edie (Evanston, IL: Northwestern University Press, 1964), 146.

44. In many respects, it is similar to Japanese philosopher Watsuji Tetsuro's reminder to us that we exist indelibly "in-between" all there is—nature, climate,

humans. This in-betweenness, *aidagara*, invokes an inescapable relation we have with each other. Watusji's notion is nothing new. It reflects a longstanding Buddhist belief in our innate interconnectedness that annihilates my illusion of an independent self.

45. Emmanuel Levinas, *Entre Nous: Thinking of the Other*, trans. Michael B. Smith and Barbara Harshav (New York: Columbia University Press, 1998), 57.

46. Salomon Malka, *Emmanuel Levinas: His Life and Legacy*, trans. Michael Kigel and Sonja M. Embree (Pittsburgh, PA: Duquesne University Press, 2006), xxiii–xxiv.

47. Richard Selzer, *The Whistler's Room: Stories and Essays* (Washington, DC: Shoemaker & Hoard, 2004), 143.

48. Emmanuel Levinas, "Meaning and Sense," in *Collected Philosophical Papers*, trans. Alphonso Lingis (Pittsburgh, PA: Duquesne University Press, 1987), 95; cited in Hagi Kenaan, *The Ethics of Visuality: Levinas and the Contemporary Gaze*, trans. Batya Stein (London: I.B. Tauris & Co., Ltd. 2013), 32.

49. Michael C. Brannigan, "Resuscitating Embodied Presence in Healthcare: the Encounter with *le Visage* in Levinas," in *Phenomenology of Bioethics: Technoethics and Lived-Experience*, ed. Susan Ferrarello (Cham, Switzerland: Springer, 2021), 140.

50. Takeshi Kimura, "Masahiro Mori's Buddhist Philosophy of Robot," *Paladyn, Journal of Behavioral Robotics* 9, no. 1 (May 5, 2018): 76. https://www.degruyter.com/document/doi/10.1515/pjbr-2018-0004/html.

51. Sherry Turkle, *Reclaiming Conversation: The Power of Talk in a Digital Age* (New York: Penguin Press, 2015), 339, 351.

Chapter Five

Poise

Should a future species glimpse at our brief history it will wonder how such strange, ant-like creatures brought about their undoing. It comes down to unheeded warnings. Take Pandora's Jar. Epimetheus ignored Prometheus' caution against accepting gifts from the gods. Although Hesiod does not describe Pandora being warned against opening the jar, tradition has somehow included that. And there is the tale of Daedalus and his son Icarus. Daedalus, believed by Athenians to be descended from the divine engineer Hephaestus, designed wings for himself and his son Icarus to escape from the labyrinth at Crete and fly away. After gluing together bird feathers with beeswax, he warned his son to fly neither too high nor too low. The young and impetuous Icarus, completely beguiled by the thrill of the moment and seized with the conceit of his new-found power over nature, ignored his father's instructions, flew too close to the sun, and paid the price, plummeting into the sea as his waxed wings melted.[1] Unheeded warnings.

One morning in early April 2020, residents of Jalandhar in the northern Indian state of Punjab woke up to witness for the first time in decades the peaks of the Dhauladhar Himalayan mountain range, nearly 120 miles away.

Air pollution in India is one of the world's worst, killing over 1.2 million people per year. In November 2019, after the air quality index (AQI) level in Delhi surpassed 800, three times the "hazardous" level, the government declared a public health emergency. The pandemic's ensuing lockdowns and long pauses in air traffic, automobile congestion, and manufacturing plants led to an historic reduction of air pollution, not only in India, but in parts of China, the Middle East, and Italy. And with dolphins spotted swimming in the Sardinian port of Cagliari, the cessation of human busyness has kindled an awakening in the natural environment, bearing witness to a fitting twist of fate: human misery accompanied by nature's healing recovery.[2] This interlude from our human intrusion in the environment, our unnatural manipulation of the natural world, and from arrogant flaunting of technological progress has led to the magnificent cinema of a sunrise. Up to now, we have lost our way without even knowing it. It took a global crisis of unsurpassed human tragedy to remind us of what really matters. Our pandemic is far from over, but have we learned our lesson thus far, and if so, for how long? Witnessing the grand Himalayan peaks, dolphins, and other natural wonders gave us a breather we so desperately needed. One long enough to wonder whether we can regain some measure of poise in our human-and-device world. The only way we can find this stability is by facing a plain truth. We need to recognize a tool for what it is—a tool. A means to an end. When it becomes more than that, when it turns into its own end, we witness the beginning of our own demise as we quietly dissolve into becoming tools of our tools.

Even after the pandemic, and we will no doubt face more, we will continue to engage with our machines and screens. Take robots. It seems they were made for these crises. Soon after it became obvious that COVID-19 would become a global scourge, a Tokyo hotel was converted to house "guests" with mild symptoms. The humanoid robot Pepper, wearing a face mask, worked as a receptionist and greeted them offering good cheer, encouragement, and reminding them to eat healthy, avoid alcohol, and keep their physical distance. The Multinational company SoftBank's Pepper provided a form of mental support for those quarantined at the hotel. And equipped with its "emotion engine," Pepper could read faces and respond to human touch. The hotel also used a robot to clean and disinfect its lobby and hallways. Pepper and other robots freed up doctors to do their work and monitor regular test data and results.[3] Throughout the contagion, robots were used to take vital signs, disinfect, and deliver food. In Wuhan, robots helped monitor patients, serve meals, and take patients' temperatures in its makeshift hospital. In Thailand, Singapore, and Israel robots assisted in monitoring and delivering meals. And in the U.S., Xenex Disinfection Services LightStrike robots were deployed in over 500 healthcare facilities to deactivate possible contamination and destroy the SARS-CoV-2 virus in various settings and hallways.[4] And we described the therapeutic, "healing" (*iyashi*) benefits of robot companions like Paro.

Robots are coming to the rescue. But remember Xiaoyi, China's AI robot that became the first of its species to pass the country's medical license exam? Think about that. It speaks volumes about what we require of doctors. If a robot can measure up to what is required to be a doctor, what does this say about the standards we set for ourselves? Have we lowered the bar? Our intellectual life has atrophied significantly in past decades due to an abundant array of forces: our growing addiction to technology as our magic fix for all problems, the churning populist illusion of crowd wisdom, a denigration of expertise (now we are all "experts"), higher education's betrayal of its mission to truly enrich the blending and balance of mind and heart and cultivating of critical thinking, etc. Neil Postman saw this happening nearly forty years ago. Contrasting the Orwellian tyranny in *1984* with Aldous Huxley's *Brave New World*, he sums up our predicament.

> Orwell warns that we will be overcome by an externally imposed oppression. But in Huxley's vision, no Big Brother is required to deprive people of their autonomy, maturity, and history. As he saw it, people will come to love their oppression, *to adore the technologies that undo their capacities to think.*[5] *(author emphasis)*

Endlessly distracted, pursuing entertainment in place of truth, we orbit the screen-altar as our universe. Screen reading no longer complements deep-reading a book. It becomes our primary text. English professor Mark Bauerlein drives home the point in his critique of higher education, challenging us to wonder, "once the Web dominates a student's intellectual sphere, does it change value, sliding into a destructive temptation to eschew more disciplined courses of thinking, to avoid reading a long poem line by line, tracking a logical argument point by point, assembling a narrative event by event?[6] When the screen replaces the imagination, learning is an uphill Sisyphean climb. An idolatry of our tools also brings about the malignant illusion of our own self-made expertise. Instead of being the commencement of life-long learning, obtaining the degree in and of itself becomes the endpoint of learning, the ultimate goal of going to college and university.

The culprit is not ignorance. That is too easy. Rather, it is an attitude, a pervasive cultural mindset, a worldview that has little to do with the world but all about "me." It is a worldview that, in the flush of societal relativism, holds that "my view" is just as true as anyone else's. International affairs expert Tom Nichols call this twisted sense of autonomy a "new Declaration of Independence." In this new Declaration, "no longer do we hold *these* truths to be self-evident, we hold *all* truths to be self-evident, even the ones that are not true. All things are knowable and every opinion on any subject is as good as any other."[7] Will we now outsource critical thinking and emotional intelligence to machines? Despite incredible benefits, our interfacing with robots opens a Pandora's Jar of perils. At heart, key concerns center on the nature and dynamic of our interfacing. Bots still have a long way to go before coming close to behaving, thinking, and feeling like humans. Even if they can simulate human facial expressions, there is little evidence that these in truth represent a person's inner state. The major misgiving in our human-robot interaction has to do not with bots, but with us—our needs, desires, values, and what we strive to become. Much hinges upon *how* we view and relate to our machines and, consequentially, with each other. Melvin Kranzberg's First Law of technology is germane: Technologies *per se* are neither good, bad, nor indifferent.[8] In effect, they are all three. Our interfacing with our machines is a collaborative recital in a chemistry shaping the dance. Its chemistry transcends the sum of the participants. Our fate rests upon how we humans dance our parts, how we use our tools and relate to them. Will we achieve that necessary balance and poise in how we interact with our machines? Pursuing this poise is imperative, morally and existentially.

Why do we use the term "poise"? Poise conveys a dignified symmetry, balance, stability, and self-control, the dance's composure of exertion and grace. In this final chapter, we address how we can sensibly pursue such poise not only in how we interact with robots but more generally in our human-to-machine engagement, because how we interface with our devices—they need not be robots—sets the tone for how we relate to ourselves and to each other. Can we humans achieve poise with our machines so that they supplement, not replace, our caregiving in ways that free us up to become better caregivers and enhance our ability to be more present with each other?

POISE THROUGH MORAL DESIGN

Pursuing poise must first address issues surrounding machine design. Machine design is distinct from a machine's moral status. Questions regarding the moral status of robots generate a whole set of concerns and complexities beyond the scope of this work. These rest upon what we can call the "plus equation," a step further from Byron Reeves and Clifford Nass' "media equation," or tendency to attribute human qualities to objects, for instance when we impulsively apply human codes of conduct to the computer.[9] In our "plus equation," if the caring robot is *more* than a mere object, since it performs caring tasks and "shows" that it cares, does that *per se* bestow a moral status? I believe that it does to a degree, in the sense of proscribing humans from intentionally misusing, abusing, and exploiting the robot. This is not because of any "harm" to the robot, but because such acts implicitly incur a moral injury upon ourselves. As I have stressed throughout, how we interact with robots says much about ourselves. In our Promethean bid to recreate ourselves, our human-robot interaction exposes our human drama, narcissism, and hubris. Whether we *can* design the perfect human, though technically spurious, heats up the more important question—Should we even make the attempt? Though this question is undoubtedly most important, we need to be pragmatic. We are already running full pace ahead in developing and designing robots. They will be a significant part of our lives. And globally, we simply do not have enough human caregivers. Furthermore, not all caregivers offer the comfort and care for the ones in need. Caregiving is life's hardest task, particularly abrasive in family relationships. Despite good intentions, we humans have only so much patience to dole out. Elder abuse remains particularly rampant among family. Ultimately, whether caregiving comes from a human or a machine, the two do not mutually exclude each other. The caring robot can nicely supplement the work and caring of the human caregiver. Morally, aside from questions of robot moral status and sentience, our main focus for now lies in our *perception* of them and how we behave accordingly. To begin, we first acknowledge the need for a morally sound robot design.

Aimee Van Wynsberghe thoughtfully takes this up through suggesting a morally sensitive framework. She grounds her discussion by way of a "value-sensitive design" (VSD) that starts with the crucial premise of technology's non-neutrality.[10] I discussed earlier this absence of value-neutrality in certain technologies in the context of our excessive attachment to devices. Values are already lodged into the design of certain technologies like assault rifles, drone bombers, computers, iPhones, and, of course, caring robots. With caring robots, it is crucial that their design and use incorporates their aims, objectives that encompass morally sound values that van Wynsberghe thoughtfully lays out. These standards offer a necessary framework for assessing the ethical legitimacy in design. Her framework considers the following: a) the context in which care occurs (hospital, nursing home, home, etc.); b) varieties of care involved (feeding, lifting, bathing, etc.); c) participants in the care process (nurse, patient, robot, etc.); d) types of robot (assistive, enabling, or replacement). Each of these must aim to nurture specific moral values. Van Wynsberghe applies four moral values underscored by political scientist Joan Tronto in her *Moral Boundaries*: "attentiveness, responsibility, competence and reciprocity."[11] For Tronto, attention, responsibility, competence and reciprocity remain the pulse of genuine caring. These four also require an embodied presence. Genuine presence involves my being present to, for, and with another. Caring is a healing relationship in which the caregiver offers her experience and competence *to* the person cared for, remains present *for* the other's well-being, and is always present *with* the other in an intrinsically moral partnership.

POISE THROUGH EMBRACING SINGULARITY

This presence with the other in moral partnership acknowledges that a person's condition is her own, a unique singularity that comprises genetic and family history, physiology, social, environmental, cultural, and personal voices. By "singularity," I do not mean science fiction writer Vernor Vinge's 1990s vision of artificially intelligent machines taking over human intelligence. Technology futurist Ray Kurzweil popularizes the idea in his *The Singularity Is Near: When Humans Transcend Biology*.[12] He predicts this singularity to occur in the 2040s, a catalyst to a technological rapture. Precisely defining my use of "singularity," with all its conceptual trimming, is not easy. The first literary journal to originate from a clinical setting is the *Bellevue Literary Review*. Its founder and noted physician and author Danielle Ofri tellingly captures singularity in her account of 91-year-old Leo Teitelbaum's death after he was rushed into the emergency room with a ruptured aorta from a car accident and had surgery. When Dr. Ofri met him briefly in the ICU, he suddenly coded with cardiac arrest. The code team charged to his bed and Ofri intubated him. Unresponsive, he died.

> Since Mr. Teitelbaum was a patient of one of the residents who I was covering overnight, it was my responsibility to document the code. I opened the chart gingerly, dreading the unending morass of papers that typically accompanies elderly, chronically ill patients . . .
>
> But I opened the cover and there was nothing. Nothing at all. I found myself face to face with the nakedness of an empty chart. Mr. Teitelbaum, it turned out, had only been admitted to the hospital a few hours ago. The progress notes were entirely blank—he hadn't had time to progress . . .
>
> And so I entered the very first progress note in Leo Teitelbaum's chart, entitled "Expiration Note."
>
> Called by RNs to evaluate patient. Patient unresponsive without pulse. CPR begun. Patient intubated (!). EKG revealed v-tach. Defibrillation x 4 without success. Rhythm degenerated to v-fib then asystole. Unresponsive to epinephrine and atropine. No palpable blood pressure. Code terminated after 20 minutes. Time of death: 3:27 a.m.
>
> I reread the note, abashed by its brevity. A human being had ended ninety-one years of life and these disembodied words constituted the official record. Mr. Teitelbaum had died without any family members around him. Just a group of strangers on the midnight shift . . .
>
> I apologized for being a stranger. For accompanying him through this intimate rite without never knowing how his voice sounded or what his touch was like. I apologized for all the pain and chaos we had put him through during his final moments.[13]

In discounting a patient's singularity, the future of caring stands in danger of becoming far too linear, dismissing caring's highly complex, multi-dimensional nature. Caring for another living being, human or nonhuman, is an ongoing, dynamic synergy that matures as the person cared-for faces each day, each encounter, impacted by any stressful event or significant change like Mr. Teitelbaum's accident and ruptured aorta. These life-shifting events are forks in the road, small and large—not able to play the piano as well because of arthritis, no longer able to drive, losing sight or hearing, not being able to climb stairs, having to use a wheelchair, getting "meals on wheels" instead of food brought in by the kids, or being driven only to Mass on Saturday instead of the routine Sunday Mass followed by a drive along Newport's Ocean Drive—that are often unnoticed or dismissed by others yet perceived as major losses by the one cared-for. Caring needs to be attentive to these shifts, big and small. They are not picked up through an algorithm. For example, though it touts a holistic delivery through its neural network collecting vital data, can China's AI-driven iCarbonX be a sensitive enough medical assistant to pick up on these signals?[14]

Aging Humans and Ageless Robots

To get a sense of a person's singularity, what comes to mind when we think of the word "old"? How about "elder"? We no longer refer to old persons, most of whom will eventually be cared-for, as elders. We may use the descriptive "elderly" to depict an old person. In the past, however, the noun "elder" had been used to bestow an honored moral authority that comes with aging and experience. This was the case in the early civilizations of China, India, so also later for the Roman Senate and the New England Puritans. Old age acquired respect. That was in the past. Now, particularly in American culture, we confer no inherent value to growing old. In contrast, "elder" bears inscribed experiences, life's victories, failures, promises, regrets, knowledge, and wisdom. These are the badges of our personal history, a history that a carebot lacks.

Here is one intractable reason why a carebot can never replace a human caregiver. A robot does not age. We grow old; carebots are ageless. They do not undergo the life-events, interruptions, relational foibles, and medical gauntlets we humans weather. And because we have faced our share of ruts and challenges, we know to some extent what those for whom we care face. Our mutual mortality constitutes the Universal Commons, the existential soil for empathy and compassion. Persons we care for own a life history colored by the trophies and scars that come with aging, like chronic illnesses with their multimorbidities. The caring robot, ageless, is naturally age-blind when it comes to an awareness of the cared-for's journey, whereas we who care for another can relate to the other because we too have our own stories, hopes, fears, and regrets. Aging brings with it a vast iceberg of lived experience that a carebot lacks. Certain life events we undergo—divorce, retirement, death of family and friends, etc.—influence our creativity, mental alertness, and emotional health. Our injuries turn into disabilities. Carebots will not have our gear-changing hiccups from the routine that remind us of our fleeting pilgrimage in this skin we inhabit.

Aging means aging bodies. This means that caregiving, alleviating another's functional difficulties, loneliness, and existential anguish—easily our most demanding and anguishing task—requires a different set of tools from the typical biomedical apparatus of treatments, tests, procedures, and medications. Medical metrics are simply not enough for caregivers. One reason is that relying solely on the metrics minimizes the vital role of intuition. In the skill and art of diagnosis, intuition helps guide the physician's culling together the clues—symptoms, signs, medical history, current family and work situations, travel, etc. Intuition has ancient roots, respected in early tribal traditions and a core feature in Asian philosophies. It was the great 16th century German physician Paracelsus who, in describing necessary qualities of a physician, included "intuition which is necessary to understand the patient, his body, his disease. He must have the feel and touch which make it possible for him to be in sympathetic communication with the patient's spirit."[15] As Paracelsus states, "to be in sympathetic communication with the patient's spirit." Will a carebot have this capacity for "sympathetic communication with the patient's spirit"? Fostering this intuition is not easy when all forces shout out "It's All In The Numbers." An excessive reliance on our heavy medical armamentarium and pharmaceuticals reflects a lack of real human clinical skill. A carebot will not have the kind of wisdom that only comes with aging and experience. Ageless, it will not learn the lessons that come with experience, mistakes, success, failure, and growth that come with imperfection. Consider medications. Medications are a mixed blessing, but for elders who endure what Arthur Kleinman calls the blight of chronicity, they can be lethal as well as life-saving. The standards of medical care for younger adults without chronic illness are shifted for elders who have to deal with wrong medications, adverse drug interaction, unknown side-effects, and an impractical regimen. Will the carebot be sensitive to the impact of pills upon the user? Aging brings with it an older body, an older body with slower reactions, at more risk of falls with multiple drugs. Falls are the bane of aging and can spell hip fractures, further illness, debility, and fatality. Without aging bodies, carebots cannot know from experience about such impending threats. Without aging bodies, neither can they appreciate each person's singularity that comes with aging. We humans fail as well to acknowledge each other's singularity, our own authenticity that comes with spontaneity, a breaking out of the template. Embracing another's singularity means avoiding the conventional trap regarding what we expect from the 'natural' order. When it comes to caring for an elder, "What do you expect? She's old." This customary snare constitutes a human sacrilege and desecrates her singularity. For the natural order is not the moral order. As noted geriatrician and author Louise Aronson wisely asserts, "Where we get into trouble is when we use this natural order of things—people shouldn't die young; dying old is our best option—as a reason *not to care* and, in medicine, not to provide the best possible care for old people."[16]

Humans share the existential pilgrimage of aging. We take part in the quest to find our place in the world. We ask questions of *what*, *where*, and *why*. We become philosophers the moment we experience a loss—of a pet, a family member, a friend—and ask *why*? Loss disrupts the comfort of the familiar, of feeling at home. And from that moment on, we seek our place. I grew up in a neighborhood in Newport, Rhode Island, known as the Fifth Ward. My Irish cousins from my grandfather's side live in the small town of Swinford, in County Mayo, western Ireland. Whereas the Fifth Ward has many streets and intersections, when I last visited Swinford, it had only few roads. Growing up in the Fifth ward and traveling abroad, I learned that place has nothing to do with intersecting streets and roads. Place is about the intersecting of lives and stories. Because of our gear-changing events, whether we shift up or slow down, we learn lessons in hardship and survival. Aging is a long drawn-out workshop on resilience as we sing, dance, struggle, pray, and mourn together. Elders have taught us about resilience, respect, civility, responsibility, and giving. They have relentlessly saved us from ourselves. The most priceless lesson we can learn from those for whom we care is knowing the meaning of "enough."[17] With our robot caring for us, who will teach us about "enough"? Who will save us from ourselves? Because we share our aging, we can relate to those for whom we care. Carebots cannot.

POISE THROUGH EMBODIED PRESENCE

The secret to pursuing poise is breathtakingly simple, yet so profoundly difficult. It lies in cultivating presence, an embodied presence, being-there-with-and-for-the-other. Through being present for another, embodied presence is inherently communicative. We never *not* communicate. The other person may or may not detect our signals, but we send them all the same through our bodies, intended or not—posture, gesture, faces, eyes, touch, voice, hands, etc. We exude these signals through living flesh. Carebots do not. And patients, residents, and others in need of care pick up on such signals. Abraham Verghese writes fluently about presence.

> Being with patients, being *present* and willing to engage directly in the manner they most want is a form of risk. The representation of the patient in the EMR (the iPatient, as I call it) is necessary. But being with the iPatient too long is a guaranteed way of *not* being present with the actual patient. It can even begin to

feel safer and simpler to be present with one of the many "enchanted objects" around us—computer screens, tablets, and smartphones—than with human beings . . . There are a few things that are timeless in medicine, unchanged since antiquity, which we can keep front and center as we bring about reform. One is the simple truth that patients want us to be more present. We as physicians want to be more present with the patient, as well, because without that contact, our professional life loses much of its meaning.

It is a one-word rallying cry for patients and physicians, the common ground we share, the one thing we should not compromise, the starting place to begin reform, the single word to put on the placard as we rally for the cause.

Presence.

Period.[18]

Listening

There is far too much noise in the world. In being present with and for the other, caregivers must first learn the skill and art of listening, a skill we *all* need to nourish. Listening is not simply hearing. That is passive, submissive. Listening must be active. It demands all our senses. Not just our ears. The person who is cared-for is a rich, complex story bundled together with plots, subplots, and intrigues uncovered and hidden, a labyrinth of Daedalus' mazes within mazes. In his novel *The Maze Maker*, Michael Ayrton's protagonist Daedalus explains the conundrum of our labyrinths.

> Each man's life is a labyrinth at the center of which lies his death, and even after death it may be that he passes through a final maze before it is all ended for him. Within the great maze of a man's life are many smaller ones, each seemingly complete in itself, and in passing through each one he dies in part, for in each he leaves behind him a part of his life and it lies dead behind him. It is a paradox of the labyrinth that its center appears to be the way to freedom.[19]

A person's journey through life's mazes unfolds in ways that can only be discerned through our fully being-with that person. It is a journey we all share. And because of this we can detect part of the "saying" that is unsaid. True listening hears what is not spoken, veiled messages spoken through the body.

It is not uncommon that the initial complaint a patient presents to a doctor—chest pain, headaches, numbing of the fingers, etc.—is not the real problem. The real problem is layered away, discovered only through attentive listening or that chance "by the way" just when the patient leaves, what my doctor John O'Leary calls the "doorknob message." The presenting complaint is the admission ticket for the appointment. In our Fourth Industrial Age of Big Data, Robotics, and AI fine-tuning to near-perfect precision its mountains of information to produce unmatched exactitude in solving the "Riddle" of diagnosis and prognosis, listening is a lost art. Even with its astounding capacity to churn through vast storehouses of data, AI "listening" cannot answer the Riddle. Genuine listening points us in the right direction. It affects what we choose to do with all this data, how to tailor it according to how well we know the person in front of us who is the patient. We also should listen to our formidable teachers from the past. Whether attributed to Hippocrates or William Osler or others, "It is more important to know what sort of person has disease than to know what sort of disease a person has" bears the wisdom of the past. Yet how easily we forget. How easily our attention is seduced by all the trappings, the novelty. How easily we become distracted by the means to the end so that the means becomes the end. How easily we lose sight of medicine's *telos*, the end for which it exists. And achieving this end, serving its ultimate purpose, is a good-in-itself. Renowned pioneer in medical ethics, the late Edmund D. Pellegrino, who devoted his life-work in the spirit of realizing this end, describes this teleological drive as the principal ground of medicine.

> A teleological oriented philosophy of medicine is certainly not a doctor-or a patient-defined entity . . . Rather, physicians do what they do and patients act as they do because both are pursuing an end in which they are joined by the realities of being ill, being healed, and professing to heal. The moral pursuit of these relationships is what determines what is right and good.[20]

The end of medicine is to heal, hopefully cure, and never stop caring. Only when healthcare ethics and its manifestations in the interdisciplinary field of bioethics keeps a firm grip on medicine's *telos* can its moral foundations be nurtured and preserved. Pellegrino reminds us of this particularly in reference to bioethics.

> So far as bioethics is concerned, I appreciate its interdisciplinary nature. But if ethics is to be normative, it must be justified by ethical argumentation, not by descriptive disciplines only. In the relationships among the disciplines of bioethics, moral philosophy remains the guiding principle. Without it, as is increasingly the case today, "ethics" in bioethics is so severely attenuated as to be on the verge of disappearance.[21]

All this demands that caregivers sculpt the art of listening, listening that nurtures and is nurtured by an embodied presence, being-there. Listening and embodied presence form a symbiotic ballet. At the same time, *being where we are and with whom we are* is our most profoundly difficult challenge as we drown in seas of distraction. Only through being there with another, letting go of the script in our heads and having "listening eyes" can we allow the door to open to see and feel through the eyes of the person who is cared for. This embodied presence is the foundation for the possibility of empathy.

Empathy

The human world is a mediated one. Our relation with the Other is via something else as a ground of shared interest. Empathy requires leaping into the Other's world by deliberately stepping outside of our own. However, carebots have no world from which they step. On this count alone, the affective reciprocity we find in human-to-human interaction does not occur with them. They no doubt pose a physical presence and, to a degree, a social one as they interact with us. But because a carebot has no world of its own—private history, story, memories, etc.—and no real interest in the wider world, it lacks the capacity for the inter-presence that occurs among humans.

As we engage more with robots, what Dumouchel and Damiano call "human-robot coevolution," with what, then, does an elder interact?[22] How genuine is one's interaction with a machine? Admittedly, those cared-for can always question the genuineness of their human caregivers so that we again stress the moral imperative of empathy. The relation between the caregiver and the person cared-for is defined and sculpted by empathy. Empathy—that over-used, misused, and abused term—is absolutely necessary in caring. How can we care for and care about someone unless we ourselves feel, at least to some degree though never identically, that person's anxiety, suffering, and needs? Empathy is neither one-dimensional nor unilateral. Rather, it dynamically infuses the relation, proven to bring about positive health outcomes. And empathy is not outcome-driven. There is no algorithm for empathy, no formula to ease another's pain and stress. Empathy is its own end, the expression of which makes us human, a reminder of who we are. This interactive dynamic can only come about through embodied presence.

My dear friends the late Doctors Marjorie and William Sirridge knew this to be the real formula in healthcare, inspiring them to establish the visionary University of Missouri-Kansas City (UMKC) Office of Medical Humanities and Bioethics in 1992. UMKC already had an unmistakably innovative School of Medicine curriculum in its 6-year combined BA/MD with its docent program of student teams led by a practicing physician so that students, from the start, acquire first-hand experience with patients, their most important teachers. The Medical Humanities and Bioethics curriculum included courses in literature, law, visual arts, music, bioethics, medical history, and cultural diversity. For example, a team consisting of a physician, art historian, and humanities specialist would teach the course "Body Image in Medicine and the Arts." Arts and humanities indispensably complements and enriches students' training in clinical skills, diagnosis, care treatment and management, and preventive medicine. They are absolutely vital. Under the leadership of its ever-caring, steadfast director, nurse, and law professor Marlyn Pesto, the office thrived as faculty believed personally and professionally in its core message: Healing in truth demands embodied presence with our patient, the whole patient. Only then can we empathize with our patients. Only through breaking out of our formulaic medical universe can we acknowledge the world of the patient and cultivate empathy. The Office of Medical Humanities and Bioethics was one of its kind, living up to Shakespeare's enduring words spoken by Portia in *The Merchant of Venice*:

> The quality of mercy is not strain'd,
> It droppeth as the gentle rain from heaven
> Upon the place beneath: it is twice blest,
> It blesseth him that gives and him that takes.[23]

Daniel Hall-Flavin, Mayo Clinic psychiatrist and former graduate of UMKC, writes of this in the context of Shakespeare's "quality of mercy." He eloquently acknowledges what is at stake if we are not able to enter into the world of the one who is cared-for.

> At stake in today's medical practice is the curiosity, creativity, and perseverance needed to embrace ambiguity and vulnerability in the service of self-discovery and fulfillment necessary if we are to be effective healers. *At stake today is our ability to be present.* At stake is our ability to craft a narrative of meaning and measure to listen generously in the service of hope and spiritual growth. At stake is our ability to craft a narrative of meaning and measure with the pain, suffering, and deportment of chronic illness. At stake is the personal agency of ourselves and our patients. At stake is the quiet mystery, majesty, and might of Mercy.[24]

We addressed empathy in earlier chapters, but it should be noted that empathy is also the cornerstone of trust, and caring is grounded upon trust, when we put ourselves in the hands of another. Can we fully trust our carebot? Clearly, the quality of our interacting with our robots hinges upon trusting that a bot can demonstrate dependability. That is a big step. Showing dependability and *being* dependable are not alike. Being dependable means choosing to be dependable, having the choice to not be dependable as well. Trust does not take place when the outcome is certain, a reason why trusting a caring robot is spurious. Onora O'Neill clearly makes this point. "Trust is not a response to certainty about others' future action. On the contrary, trust is needed precisely when and because we lack certainty about others' future action: it is redundant when action or outcomes are guaranteed. That is why we find it hard, as well as important, to try to place trust reasonably rather than foolishly."[25]

Touch

What more tangibly affirms embodied presence? Touch. This embodied interaction is palpably evident in human-to-human touch. The human touch can be an irreplaceable gift. Consider the physical contact between caregiver and cared-for when it comes to lifting, feeding, and bathing. Van Wynsberghe gives us a wonderful illustration of what is involved.

> When a patient is lifted by the care-giver, it is a moment in which the patient is at one of their most vulnerable. The patient trusts the care-giver and through this action a bond is formed and/or strengthened which reinforces the relationship between care-giver and the care-receiver . . . trust, bonds, and the relationship, are integral components for ensuring that the care-receiver will comply with their treatment plan, will take their medication and be honest about their symptoms.[26]

This scenario captures the existential and moral quality of flesh-to-flesh touch. So also, caring for someone by bathing him involves much more than the perfunctory and necessary motions of positioning and washing. Bathing another living being profoundly demonstrates the power of the human touch, communicating reassurance, comfort, empathy, and respect. It is saying "I am here for you" without having to say it. Touch signals caring in a threatening world. When she worked as a volunteer rape crisis counselor, Danielle Ofri recalls meeting a young homeless woman who had been raped.

> The woman was disheveled, dirty, and powerfully malodorous. My stomach churned when a roach sauntered out of her tattered dress. I didn't think I had the wherewithal to overcome my disgust to do my job.
>
> As I cringed behind the Triage desk, pretending to be involved with paperwork, a nurse's aide approached the woman. She smoothed the woman's matted hair. She took her dirt-encrusted hand and gently guided her to the shower, all the while talking softly to her with a reassuring smile. I was awed and humbled.[27]

Touch in the Saying

Touch offers a harbor of shelter, that all is well. Embracing each other before sleep sends the message that all is right with the world. Touch wears its own language and dialect, more intoxicating than words. Touch energizes comfort at a wake or funeral. Words represent the Said, Levinas' *le Dit*. It is the saying, *le dire*, that pre-conceptually occurs in the approach, exposure, and touch. Emmanuel Levinas reminds us of the seismic chasm between *Le Dit* (the Said) and *le dire* (the saying). Whereas the former denotes a static thematizing of a relation with another, the latter refers to a dynamic relation that is intrinsically moral. *Le dire* encompasses not *what* we say but *how* we express it, along with how we choose to leave it unspoken well before approaching the other. Levinas: "Saying is not a game. Antecedent to the verbal signs it conjugates, to the linguistic systems and the semantic glimmerings, a foreword preceding languages, it is the proximity of one to the other, the commitment of an approach, the one for the other, the very signifying-ness of signification."[28] "Saying is not a game." It is not reducible to mere linguistics nor captured in dense objectification or concepts. Saying is serious business, for it is the condition for an encounter with the other that compels moral responsibility. In this self-exposure before the other, the body speaks its own fertile language so that the saying occurs in the context of our proximity, initiating an embodied presence and approach to the other, of necessity our neighbor by virtue of proximity. For instance, our preference for texting over speaking and certainly over face-to-face engagement, can be a symptom of our desire to avoid the risks and uncertainties in an inter-presence with the other. We prefer the security of the Said and bestow upon it an unmerited primacy. Saying, however, naturally risky, constitutes the ground of our being-for-the-other. It affirms the priority of ethics over ontology. Moral responsibility precedes ontic status through *le dire* which "weaves an intrigue of responsibility."[29] Levinas personally endured the annihilation of moral responsibility throughout his dehumanizing war ordeal. Even worse, most of his family were murdered along with millions during Shoah. Yet his resilient hope spurs him on to powerfully assert the moral gravity that abides in our encounter with the other.

> Saying states and thematizes the said, but signifies it to the other, a neighbor, with a signification that has to be distinguished from that borne by words in the said. This signification to the other occurs in proximity. Proximity is quite distinct from every other relationship, and has to be conceived as a responsibility for the other; it might be called humanity, or subjectivity, or self. Being and entities weigh heavily by virtue of the saying that gives them light. Nothing is more grave, more august, than responsibility for the other, and saying, in which there is no play, has a gravity more grave than its own being or not being.[30]

The saying represents *how* we are there and *how* we offer ourselves in being present. Touch is our most important sense, our oxygen for reaching out.[31]

Touch transmits energy, a life force. It is electric. The gentle clasp of our hand on another's shoulder conducts human warmth. It is subtle, harmless, faint, without motive, yet makes all the difference. Touch offers comfort even when it does not come from a living human. There is no denying that our pets and other animals surely convey comfort and calm. Like the real nightingale in Hans Christian Andersen's tale, they are living beings, not programmed machines wound up to sing. They often sense our own anxieties in ways that enable us to feel more connected with them than with humans. Their fidelity to us is without condition. This power of touch through our pets demonstrates how this power works both ways. We comfort the pet just as our pet comforts us.

Again, this is about context, not just content. In a home setting, for reasons of dignity and privacy, a wife may not wish her husband to bath or lift her and may prefer instead a robot.[32] This is similar to why many humans prefer sharing their most intimate thoughts and feelings with a machine, a chatbot, rather than with a human. This makes sense as a face-saving way to avoid further shame and embarrassment. She views the robot's value in its instrumentality, and holds on to her dignity. At the same time, this does not diminish the richness of the human touch. *There is no substitute for the human touch.* The human touch—lifting, bathing, etc.—offers a silent, soft bond. Through bodily intuitiveness, touch enables that all-important trust on the part of the cared-for. We always return full circle to that perennial lesson in healthcare: Healing is not only about cure, but *always* about care. The difference one letter makes. Context/content, care/cure. Caring helps heal and make whole while restoring dignity. The simple act of touch is an embodied, silent conversation. Its dual-directionality does not work with caring robots.

The Lost Art of Touch in Medicine

The human touch has become a lost art in medicine. In his *The Youngest Science*, Lewis Thomas prophetically feared that a doctor's real work, to care for the sick, "might be replaced with looking after machines." He witnessed medicine's progress from its helplessness treating fatal diseases like tuberculosis and syphilis to amassing novel advanced technologies that could stave off death without, however, offering any quality in staying alive. Contemporary medicine's "progress" is a transition from cultivating the art of comforting the incurable to more scientific sophistication in laboring to cure the incurable. Remembering how his father, also a doctor, made house visits, talked with and touched his patients, Thomas describes touch as a doctor's most valuable tool. "The close-up, reassuring, warm touch of the physician, the comfort and concern, the long, leisurely discussions in which everything including the dog can be worked into the conversation, are disappearing from the practice of medicine, and this may turn out to be too great a loss for the doctor as well as for the patient."[33] Today this sounds archaic given how machine-like and routine medicine has become along with ever-increasing institutional pressures our doctors face. In describing how René Laennec's "cylinder," or stethoscope, became a major turning point in doctors' encounters with their patients, stepping beyond simple palpation and auscultation through creating a clinical distance via an instrument, Stanley Joel Reiser claims that the technology "reformulated the relationship between doctors and patients, through the use of an instrument that took the mantle of illness out of the hands of patients and placed it in the doctor's orbit."[34] Since then, the specificity of diagnostic techniques with their narrow focus has disregarded the dynamic singularity of the patient.

> Diagnostic technologies focus users on particular aspects of reality. The more compelling and authentic this reality seems, the greater is the user's belief that it *says enough*. In this way a partial perspective of a complex reality becomes an acceptable substitute for the whole. Thus, if the sound tells all, why bother with what the person thinks or feels?[35]

In Closing

There are no accidents. When Icarus plunged into the sea after ignoring his father's warning, his downfall was the inevitable outcome of his obsession with his wings, his pride, illusion of power, *hubris*, and lack of self-awareness. In *The Maze Maker*, Daedalus tells us about his son.

> Icarus was always in combat, with other men, with bulls, with horses, with himself, and I, heedless, remained in combat with intractable substances and difficult materials. I love order and measured harmony. The proper conquest is to me the conquest implicit in the making of a satisfactory image or a tool which suits its function. I need no other power. Icarus needed power and although I am proud, his pride eclipsed mine. He was, as I say, a fool. He never became a man although he became an immortal. I do not think he ever discovered who he was.[36]

It remains to be seen what our human-machine interface bodes for the future. How will we think of our wings? How will that affect how we think of ourselves? In what ways will our human-robot interaction influence how we care for others? Will we find a reasonable symmetry, poise, and balance in our interaction with our tools? Or will we rely so thoroughly on a carebot that we delude ourselves into believing that its presence will be good enough for grandma? For dad? For our child? For ourselves? These are decisive questions for straightforward reasons. The less time we spend with each other, the worse we get at *being* with each other. We stand in danger of being so ensnared by our machines that we become more like them. In her eye-opening study of machine gambling, cultural anthropologist Natasha Dow Schüll describes Patsy, a welfare officer at a food stamp center in Nevada.

> In the simplified, mechanical exchange with gambling machines, she insulates herself from the complicated and often insurmountable needs and worries of others, to a point where she herself becomes robotlike, impervious to human distress and her inability to assuage it. "The machines were like heaven," Patsy remembers, "because I didn't have to talk to them, just feed them money." The digitized process of "feeding" and response is a form of exchange emptied of the uncertainties and inscrutabilities of social relations.[37]

So too with our computer, iPad, iPhone, TV, etc., as we climb into our screens, sucked down the rabbit hole of multi-distraction. The bold irony is that in escaping from the banal with its routine interruptions and distractions, we lose ourselves in the device of which the primary strategy is to distract. Our ultimate distraction. Our immersion in the machine offers a safe haven valorizing the screen and vaporizing time. The more we engage with our devices, the more second-nature it becomes, the easier it is to merge *into* the über-device of devices, our robot. While freeing ourselves from the humdrum and quotidian, we become further enchained. As in many marriages and partnerships, after so long, we take on the character of our companion. And if interfacing with robots demands less of us, why bother with the struggle and nuisance of human-to-human interaction? As in exercise, if we do not use it, we lose it. Our communal, give-and-take muscles atrophy.[38] If we forego caring for one another, we chisel away our humanness.

How will we relate to our wings? Though the jury is still out, we jurors deliberate every day in how we relate with people, especially those dear to us. Each day, every encounter and missed opportunity sets the key, major and minor, for our unfolding symphony. The future is not a reified "out there," not yet here. It unfurls in our every moment. Is there room for hope in this unfurling? If so, what is the quality of our hope? Recall the mystery behind Pandora closing her jar in time to seal in the spirit Hope, *elpis*. Is ours a blind hope? Or is it a reasoned hope, an ally in braving our challenge? Throughout our pandemic we hear stories of people spitting on mask-wearers, mutual intimidations, threats, and endless tiring anecdotes of opportunism and excessive entitlement. Tales of kindness stand less chance of seeing light, yet they occur. In fact, we humans tend more to show compassion during hard times despite the incessant media echo chamber force-feeding news of selfishness, violence, political acrimony, and national divisiveness. Small acts of solidarity and community do take place, acts that psychologist Jamil Zaki calls "catastrophe compassion."[39] For example, early in the pandemic, mutual aid groups sprang up throughout the U.S., Canada, Germany, and the U.K. with volunteers buying and delivering groceries and medicines to elders and those staying at home due to their health.[40]

Viruses will continue to haunt us. COVID-19 is still unraveling. There are global concerns over the more worrisome and transmissible Delta variant, B.1.617.2, having spread to more than 130 countries as of this writing.[41] It has accounted for a major surge of infections in India, and in 90 percent of recent samples in the U.K., it is no doubt the dominant variant.[42] How will we manage to coexist with new threats, including pathogens, on this planet? A dot is not just a dot. A single occurrence in one part of the world is not one isolated event. It impacts all, however minuscule, however slight. MIT meteorologist Edward Norton Lorenz made this evident over half a century earlier in his theory of the butterfly effect, how one butterfly in Brazil, by simply flapping its wings, can spark conditions for a tornado in Texas. Because of this "sensitive dependence on initial conditions," slight changes produce giant outcomes.[43] Nature's dazzling puzzle cannot be captured through the inherently imprecise quality of human metrics. On our overwhelmingly complex planet, this Daedalus labyrinth we have created for ourselves, what appears ordinary, unexceptional, and irrelevant participates in a web and flow that generates constant waves, at times tsunamis, of cause and effect. This is what Buddhist teachings have reminded us all along, this interpenetration of rising and falling, our inescapable interconnectedness.

What then is caring, this moving target, tangled and fuzzy? Because caring places special value on who or what is cared for, caring is more than simply task-oriented. Because I care for Brooke, I show her how much I care, not just tell her. Because I care for my family and friends, my caring is not only defined through those occasional cards, texts, and phone calls. Because I care for my students, my caring is not limited to just showing up for class and teaching. Caring is not merely acting in caring ways, care-acting. Caring about is distinct from caring for. Caring *about* someone depicts an attitude toward whom we care about. Caring *for* someone involves acting accordingly on behalf of whom we care about. We can care about someone without doing anything about it, without taking care of that someone. And vice versa, we can take care of someone without caring about that person. Yet, as Joan Tronto incisively reminds us, good care demands *both* caring about and caring for. Because caring is its own healing process, it is more than simply care-acting. To heal is to make whole. As with all patients who are vulnerable precisely because they are patients, the frail, particularly elders and disabled, need restoration of wholeness, reassurance, calm, and, most importantly, dignity.

In closing, imagine a caring robot in a nursing home who acts as a music therapist for residents. The carebot is care-acting, going to each room, programmed to play any kind of music occupants would like to hear. The carebot asks each resident his or her music choice and immediately downloads and plays the music. This is healing in many ways. Music pulls us in. Listening to music is intensely active and experiential; its melody and cadence engages us physically, emotionally, and sensually. "Without music, life would be an error," writes Nietzsche.[44] Music is the major artery to a person's spirit. Its ineffable rhythm draws us together. Now can this carebot replace a human caregiver who acts as a music therapist? Clinical psychologist and author Mary Pipher relates this story of Crystal, a music therapist at a nursing home.

> The main thing residents want is her time. Often people pull out scrapbooks with old pictures of their parents and families. Crystal asks questions like "What did you get in trouble for?" or "How did you meet your spouse?" She tries to focus on good stories and accomplishments. Wedding-day stories tend to be funny and happy. Sometimes she holds the residents' hands. One old man said to her, "You are my best friend."
>
> . . . Crystal noted that the people at the Manor take care of one another. They worry if their friends are not eating. Residents speak up for one another, visit the shut-ins, and send cards. They make sure Crystal plays every person's favorite song . . . These elders help her keep things in perspective. None of them has money, but the ones who are happy have people they love . . . Crystal hopes she can be like her favorite residents when she is old—good-natured and good-hearted, not a complainer.
>
> Crystal isn't a mental health professional, but she gives the gifts of touch and laughter. She doesn't give much advice, just listens to the sad stories and then encourages people to enjoy good memories.[45]

Crystal, in her person and embodied presence for others, shares her "gifts of touch and laughter" as she pushes her music cart from room to room. It is her being-there and listening as she chats with each resident and learns from them. "These elders help her keep things in perspective." Through her physical personal presence, she and those whom she visits nurture the dynamic, life-saving give-and-take of caring. It comes down to posing Aristotle's question regarding purpose, or *telos*. What is the purpose of caring? To what end is a caring robot used? To effectively perform a certain task like lifting, care-acting, the robot has enormous value. To offer real care, however, demands more. Genuine care is a landscape that only humans can navigate with their humble backpack of presence.

NOTES

1. Adrienne Mayor, *Gods and Robots: Myths, Machines, and Ancient Dreams of Technology* (Princeton, NJ: Princeton University Press, 2018), 75–81.

2. Sarakshi Rai, "The Himalayas are Visible from India for the First Time in 30 Years because of Covid-19 Lockdown," *Esquire, The Middle East* (April 12, 2020), https://www.esquireme.com/content/45334-the-himalayas-are-visible-from-india-for-the-first-time-in-30-years-because-of-covid-19-lockdown

3. "'I'm cheering for you': Robot Welcome at Tokyo Quarantine Hotel," *The Straits Times*, May 1, 2020, https://www.straitstimes.com/asia/east-asia/im-cheering-for-you-robot-welcome-at-tokyo-quarantine.

4. Richard Blake, "In Coronavirus Fight, Robots Report For Disinfection Duty," *Forbes*, April 17, 2020, https://www.forbes.com/sites/richblake1/2020/04/17/in-covid-19-fight-robots-report-for-disinfection-duty/?sh=1060a4a02ada.

5. Neil Postman, *Amusing Ourselves to Death: Public Discourse in the Age of Show Business* (New York: Viking Penguin, Inc., 1985), vii.

6. Mark Bauerlein, *The Dumbest Generation: How the Digital Age Stupifies Young Americans and Jeopardizes Our Future* (New York: Jeremy P. Tarcher/Penguin, 2008), 141.

7. Tom Nichols, *The Death of Expertise: The Campaign against Established Knowledge and Why It Matters* (New York: Oxford University Press, 2017), xi.

8. Melvin Kranzberg, "Technology and History: Kranzberg's Laws," *Technology and Culture* 27, no. 3 (July 1986): 547, https://doi.org/10.2307/3105385.

9. Bryon Reeves and Clifford Nass, *The Media Equation: How People Treat Computers, Television, and New Media Like Real People and Places* (Stanford, CA: Center for the Study of Language and Information, Stanford University, 2003).

10. Aimee van Wynsberghe, "Designing Robots for Care: Care Centered Value-Sensitive Design," *Science and Engineering Ethics* 19 (2013): 407–33, DOI: 10.1007/s11948-011-9343-6.

11. Joan Tronto, *Moral Boundaries: A Political Argument for an Ethic of Care* (New York: Routledge, 1993), cited in van Wynsberghe, "Designing Robots for Care," 411.

12. Ray Kurzweil, *The Singularity Is Near: When Humans Transcend Biology* (New York: Penguin Books, 2006).

13. Danielle Ofri, *Singular Intimacies: Becoming a Doctor at Bellevue* (New York: Penguin Books, 2003), 136–37.

14. Eric Topol, *Deep Medicine: How Artificial Intelligence Can Make Healthcare Human Again* (New York: Basic Books, 2019), 271.

15. Cited in Bernard Lown, *The Lost Art of Healing* (New York: Ballantine Books, 1996), 3.

16. Louise Aronson, *Elderhood: Redefining Aging, Transforming Medicine, Reimagining Life* (New York: Bloomsbury Publishing Inc., 2019), 367.

17. Mary Pipher, *Another Country: Navigating the Emotional Terrain of Our Elders* (New York: Riverhead Books, 1999), 89.

18. Abraham Verghese, "The Importance of Being," *Health Affairs* 35, no. 10 (October 2016): 1926–27.

19. Michael Ayrton, *The Maze Maker* (Chicago, IL: University of Chicago Press, 1967), 12.

20. Edmund D. Pellegrino, "Philosophy of Medicine: Should It Be Teleologically or Socially Constructed?" in *The Philosophy of Medicine Reborn: A Pellegrino Reader*, ed. H. Tristam Englehardt, Jr. and Fabrice Jotterand (Notre Dame, IN: Notre Dame University Press, 2008), 53.

21. Edmund D. Pellegrino, "Apologia for a Medical Truant," in *The Philosophy of Medicine Reborn: A Pellegrino Reader*, ed. H. Tristam Englehardt, Jr. and Fabrice Jotterand (Notre Dame, IN: Notre Dame University Press, 2008), xv.

22. Paul Dumouchel and Luisa Damiano, *Living with Robots*, trans. Malcolm DeBevoise (Cambridge, MA: Harvard University Press, 2017), 167.

23. Cited in Daniel K. Hall-Flavin, "The Quality of Mercy," in *Spirituality and Deep Connectedness: Views on Being Fully Human*, ed. Michael C. Brannigan (Lanham, MD: Lexington Books, 2018), 52.

24. Hall-Flavin, "The Quality of Mercy," 61.

25. Onora O'Neill, *Autonomy and Trust in Bioethics* (Cambridge, UK: Cambridge University Press, 2002), 13.

26. van Wynsberghe, "Designing Robots for Care," 417.

27. Ofri, *Singular Intimacies*, 169.

28. Emmanuel Levinas, *Otherwise Than Being or Beyond Essence*, trans. Alphonso Lingis (Pittsburgh, PA: Duquesne University Press, 1998), 5.

29. Levinas, *Otherwise Than Being*, 6.

30. Levinas, *Otherwise Than Being*, 46.

31. Diane Ackerman, *A Natural History of the Senses* (New York: Random House, Inc., Vintage Books, 1990), 77–78.

32. van Wynsberghe, "Designing Robots for Care," 425.

33. Lewis Thomas, *The Youngest Science: Notes of a Medicine-Watcher* (New York: The Viking Press, 1983), 57.

34. Stanley Joel Reiser, *Technological Medicine: The Changing World of Doctors and Patients* (New York: Cambridge University Press, 2009), 7–8.

35. Reiser, *Technological Medicine*, 12–13.

36. Ayrton, *The Maze Maker*, 92.

37. Natasha Dow Schüll, *Addiction by Design: Machine Gambling in Las Vegas* (Princeton, NJ: Princeton University Press, 2012), 195–96.

38. Noreena Hertz, *The Lonely Century: How to Restore Human Connection in a World That's Pulling Apart* (New York: Currency, 2021).

39. Jamil Zaki, "Catastrophe Compassion: Understanding and Extending Prosociality Under Crisis," *Trends in Cognitive Sciences* 24, no. 8 (August 2020): 587–89.

40. Sigal Samuel, "How to Help People during the Pandemic, One Google Spreadsheet at a Time," *Vox*, April 16, 2020, https://www.vox.com/future-perfect/2020/3/24/21188779/mutual-aid-coronavirus-covid-19-volunteering.

41. United Nations, "COVID-19 Infections Rse, Delta Variant Spreads to 132 Countries," *UN News*, July 28, 2021, https://news.un.org/en/story/2021/07/1096572.

42. Stephen Fidler and Suryatapa Bhattacharya, "The Delta Covid-19 Variant Is Spreading: What Does This Mean for the US?" *Wall Street Journal*, June 18, 2021, https://www.wsj.com/articles/delta-variant-covid-19-11620722888?tesla=y.

43. Peter Dizikes, "When the Butterfly Effect Took Flight," *MIT Technology Review*, Feb. 22, 2011, https://www.technologyreview.com/2011/02/22/196987/when-the-butterfly-effect-took-flight/.

44. Friedrich Nietzsche, *Twilight of the Idols Or, How to Philosophize with a Hammer*, trans. Richard Polt (Indianapolis, IN: Hackett Publishing Company, Inc., 1997), 10.

45. Pipher, *Another Country*, 197–98.

Bibliography

Ackerman, Diane. *A Natural History of the Senses*. New York: Random House, Inc., Vintage Books, 1990.
AI in Healthcare, Summer 2018. https://www.purestorage.com/content/dam/pdf/en/thought-leadership/protected/tl-ai-in-healthcare-article.pdf.
AliveCor. "FDA Grants First-Ever Clearances to Detect Bradycardia and Tachycardia on a Personal ECG Device." *Cision PR Newswire*, Apr. 23, 2019. https://www.prnewswire.com/news-releases/fda-grants-first-ever-clearances-to-detect-bradycardia-and-tachycardia-on-a-personal-ecg-device-300835949.html.
Al-Lamee, Rasha, David Thompson, Hakim-Moulay Dehbi, Sayan Sen, Kare Tang, John Davies, Thomas Keeble et al. "Percutaneous Coronary Intervention in Stable Angina (ORBITA): A Double-Blind Randomized Controlled Trial." *The Lancet* 391, no. 10115 (Jan. 6, 2018): 31–40. https://doi.org/10.1016/S0140-6736(17)32714-9.
American Nurses Association. "What Is Nursing?" Accessed Feb. 6, 2020. https://www.nursingworld.org/practice-policy/workforce/what-is-nursing.
Anders, Günther. *L'obsolescence de l'homme: Sur l'âme à l'époque de la deuxième revolution industrielle*. Translated by Christophe David. Paris: Ivrea, 2001.
Angelucci, Adriano, Pierluigi Graziani and Maria Grazia Rossi. "The Uncanny Valley: A Working Hypothesis." In *Social Robots: Boundaries, Potential, Challenges*, edited by Marco Nørskov, 123–37. Surrey, UK: Ashgate Publishing Limited, 2016.
Aronson, Louise. *Elderhood: Redefining Aging, Transforming Medicine, Reimagining Life*. New York: Bloomsbury Publishing Inc., 2019.
Asimov, Isaac. *Robots and Empire*. Garden City, NY: Doubleday, 1985.
Asimov, Isaac. "Runaround." *Astounding Science Fiction*, March, 1942: 94–103.
Ayrton, Michael. *The Maze Maker*. Chicago, IL: University of Chicago Press, 1967.
Barcaro, Roseangela, Martina Mazzoleni, and Paolo Virgili. "Ethics of Care and Robot Caregivers." *Prolegomena* 17, no. 1 (2018): 71–80. doi:10.26362/20180204.
Barsky, Benjamin A., Eric Reinhart, Paul Farmer, and Salmaan Keshavje. "Vaccination plus Decarceration—Stopping Covid-19 in Jails and Prisons." *The New England Journal of Medicine* 384 (April 29, 2021): 1583–85.
Bauerlein, Mark. *The Dumbest Generation: How the Digital Age Stupifies Young Americans and Jeopardizes Our Future*. New York: Jeremy P. Tarcher/Penguin, 2008.

Becker, Ernest. *The Denial of Death*. New York: The Free Press, 1973.
Blake, Richard. "In Coronavirus Fight, Robots Report for Disinfection Duty." *Forbes*, April 17, 2020. https://www.forbes.com/sites/richblake1/2020/04/17/in-covid-19-fight-robots-report-for-disinfection-duty/?sh=1060a4a02ada.
Bramsløw, Lars, and Douglas L. Beck. "Deep Neural Networks in Hearing Devices." *Hearing Review.Com*, Special Issue, Hearing Aids and Cognition, January 2021, 28–31. https://www.ilhearing.org/assets/Education/2021/Bramslow%20Beck%20-%20Deep%20Neural%20Networks%20in%20Hearing%20Devices.pdf.
Brannigan, Michael C. *Cultural Fault Lines in Healthcare: Reflections on Cultural Competency*. Lanham, MD: Lexington Books, Rowman & Littlefield, 2012.
Brannigan, Michael C. "Despite Medical Advances, Keen Attention still Required." *Albany Times Union*, September 26, 2019. https://www.timesunion.com/opinion/article/Despite-medical-advances-keen-attention-still-14471619.php.
Brannigan, Michael C. "Does Seamus the Robot Care for Me?" *Times Union*, Feb. 27, 2011. https://www.timesunion.com/opinion/article/Does-Seamus-the-robot-care-for-me-1032481.php.
Brannigan, Michael C. *Japan's March 2011 Disaster and Moral Grit: Our Inescapable In-between*. Lanham, MD: Lexington Books, 2015.
Brannigan, Michael C. "Need for Face-to-Face Contact Transcends Viral Moment." *Times Union*, May 28, 2020. https://www.timesunion.com/opinion/article/Need-for-face-to-face-contact-transcends-viral-15301656.php.
Brannigan, Michael C. "On Robots, Depression, and the Lure of the Not-Quite-Real." *Times Union*, April 1, 2021.
Brannigan, Michael C. "Resuscitating Embodied Presence in Healthcare: The Encounter with *le Visage* in Levinas." In *Phenomenology of Bioethics: Technoethics and Lived-Experience*, edited by Susan Ferrarello, 131–42. Cham, Switzerland: Springer, 2021.
Breazeal, Cynthia. *Designing Sociable Robots*. Cambridge, MA: MIT Press, 2002.
Broadbent, Elizabeth, Vinayak Kumar, Xingyan Li, John Sollers 3rd, Rebecca Q. Stafford, Bruce, A. MacDonald, and Daniel M. Wegner. "Robots with Display Screens: A Robot with a More Humanlike Face Display Is Perceived to Have More Mind and Better Personality." *Plos One* 8, no. 8 (August 28, 2013): 1–8. https://doi.org/10.1371/journal.pone.0072589.
Broadbent, Elizabeth, Rie Tamagawa, Anna Patience, Brett Knock, Ngaire Kerse, Karen Day, and Bruce A MacDonald. "Attitudes towards Health-Care Robots in a Retirement Village." *Australasia Journal of Aging* 31, no. 2 (June 2021): 115–20.
Brynjolfsson, Erik, and Andrew McAfee. *The Second Machine Age: Work, Progress, and Prosperity in a Time of Brilliant Technologies*. New York, NY: W.W. Norton Company, Inc., 2014.
Buoy Health. Accessed May 2021. https://www.buoyhealth.com/.
Burton, Thomas M. "New Stroke Technology to Identify Worst Cases Gets FDA Approval." *The Wall Street Journal*, May 30, 2018. https://www.wsj.com/articles/new-stroke-technology-to-identify-worst-cases-gets-fda-approval-1527709670.

Carr, Nicholas. *The Glass Cage. Automation and Us*. New York: W.W. Norton & Company, 2014.
Carr, Nicholas. "These Are Not the Robots We Were Promised." *New York Times*, Sept. 9, 2017. https://www.nytimes.com/2017/09/09/opinion/sunday/household-robots-alexa-homepod.html.
Cassell, Eric J. *Doctoring: The Nature of Primary Care Medicine*. Oxford: Oxford University Press, 1997.
Chabris, Christopher, and Daniel Simons. *The Invisible Gorilla: How Our Intuitions Deceive Us*. New York: Broadway Paperbacks, 2009.
Chen, M. Keith, Judith A. Chevalier, and Elisa F. Long. "Nursing Home Staff Networks and COVID-19." *PNAS, Proceedings of the National Academy of Sciences of the United States of America* 118, no. 1 (Jan. 5, 2021): 1–7. https://doi.org/10.1073/pnas.2015455118.
Chhith, Alex. "Dedicated Las Vegas Nurse with a 'Big Heart' Killed by COVID-19 at 39." *Las Vegas Review-Journal*, August 19, 2020. https://www.reviewjournal.com/local/local-las-vegas/dedicated-las-vegas-nurse-with-big-heart-killed-by-covid-19-at-39-2098596/.
Christakis, Nicholas A. *Apollo's Arrow: The Profound and Enduring Impact of Coronavirus on the Way We Live*. New York: Little, Brown Spark, 2020.
Clark, Andy. *Natural-Born Cyborgs: Minds, Technologies, and the Future of Human Intelligence*. New York: Oxford University Press, 2003.
Clark, Andy. *Supersizing the Mind: Embodiment, Action, and Cognitive Extension*. Oxford: Oxford University Press, 2011.
Clark, Andy, and David Chalmers. "The Extended Mind." *Analysis* 58, no. 1 (January 1998): 7–19.
Cohen, John. *Human Robots in Myth and Science*. London: Allen and Unwin, 1966.
Cohen, Stanley. *States of Denial: Knowing about Atrocities and Suffering*. Cambridge, UK: Polity Press, 2001.
Cole, Jessie. "Botox Silences Women's Faces—And Freezes Out Empathy in Body Language." *The Guardian*, May 22, 2013. https://www.theguardian.com/commentisfree/2013/may/22/botox-silences-womens-faces-empathy.
"COVID-19: Health Care Worker Death Toll Rises to at Least 17000 as Organizations Call for Rapid Vaccine Rollout." Amnesty International, Mar. 5, 2021. https://www.amnesty.org/en/latest/news/2021/03/covid19-health-worker-death-toll-rises-to-at-least-17000-as-organizations-call-for-rapid-vaccine-rollout/.
Csepregi, Gabor. *The Clever Body*. Calgary, Alberta, Canada: University of Calgary Press, 2006.
Dall'Agnol, Darlei. "Caring Robots." *Practical Ethics* Blog, Oxford University, June 25, 2015. http://blog.practicalethics.ox.ac.uk/2015/06/guest-post-caring-robots.
de Campos, Amisha Parekh, and Susan Daniels. "Ethical Implications of COVID-19: Palliative Care, Public Health, and Long-Term Care Facilities." *Journal of Hospice and Palliative Nursing* 23, no. 2 (April 2021): 120–27.
Deutsche, Helene. "Some Forms of Emotional Disturbance and Their Relationship to Schizophrenia." *Psychoanalytic Quarterly* 11 (1942): 301–21.

Dizikes, Peter. "When the Butterfly Effect Took Flight." *MIT Technology Review*, Feb. 22, 2011. https://www.technologyreview.com/2011/02/22/196987/when-the-butterfly-effect-took-flight/.

Dumouchel, Paul, and Luisa Damiano. *Living with Robots*. Translated by Malcolm DeBevoise. Cambridge, MA: Harvard University Press, 2017.

Eaton, Joe. "Who Is to Blame." *AARP Bulletin* 61, no. 10 (December 2020): 21–25.

Ekman, Paul. *Emotions Revealed: Recognizing Faces and Feelings to Improve Communication and Emotional Life*. New York: Henry Holt and Company, Owl Books, 2003.

"Elderly Citizens Accounted for Record 28.4% of Japan's Population in 2018, Data Show." *The Japan Times*, Sept. 15, 2019. https://www.japantimes.co.jp/news/2019/09/15/national/elderly-citizens-accounted-record-28-4-japans-population-2018-data-show/#.Xjs3XKZYZPY.

Ellul, Jacques. *The Technological Society*. Translated by John Wilkinson. New York: Knopf, 1964.

Engelbrecht, Cora, and Caroline Kim. "Zoom Shivas and Prayer Hotlines: Ultra-Orthodox Jewish Traditions Upended by Coronavirus." *New York Times*, April 16, 2020. https://www.nytimes.com/video/us/100000007061978/coronavirus-ultra-orthodox-jewish-traditions.html.

Esteva, Andre, Brett Kuprel, Roberto A. Novoa, Justin Ko, Susan M. Swetter, Helen M. Blau, and Sebastian Thrun. "Dermatologist-Level Classification of Skin Cancer with Deep Neural Networks." *Nature* 542 (Feb. 2017): 115–18. https://doi.org/10.1038/nature21056.

Feinberg, Joel. *Harm to Self*, Volume 3. New York: Oxford University Press, 1986.

Feinberg, Joel. *Harmless Wrongdoing*, Volume 4. New York: Oxford University Press, 1990.

Felts, Adam. "MIT AgeLab Hosts Governor Baker, Winners of In Good Company Challenge." MIT News, Dec. 26, 2018. https://news.mit.edu/2018/mit-agelab-hosts-governor-baker-in-good-company-challenge-winners-1226.

Ferrarello, Susan, ed. *Phenomenology of Bioethics: Technoethics and Lived-Experience*. Cham, Switzerland: Springer, 2021.

Fidler, Stephen, and Suryatapa Bhattacharya. "The Delta Covid-19 Variant Is Spreading: What Does This Mean for the US?" *Wall Street Journal*, June 18, 2021. https://www.wsj.com/articles/delta-variant-covid-19-11620722888?tesla=y.

Fischer, Jeremy, and Rachel Fredericks. "The Creeps as Moral Emotion." *Ergo* 7, no. 6 (2020), 27 pages. Available at SSRN: https://ssrn.com/abstract=3739193.

Fox, Renée C. "The evolution of medical uncertainty." *Milbank Memorial Fund Quarterly/Health and Society* 58, no. 1 (Winter 1980): 1–49.

Fox, Renée C. *Experiment Perilous: Physicians and Patients Facing the Unknown*. Glencoe, IL: Free Press, 1959.

Fox, Renée C. *In the Field: A Sociologist Journey*. New Brunswick, NJ: Transaction Publishers, 2011.

Fox, Renée C., and Judith P. Swazey. *The Courage to Fail: A Social View of Organ Transplants and Dialysis*. Chicago: University of Chicago Press, 1973.

Friedman, Batya, and Peter H. Kahn, Jr. "Human Agency and Responsible Computing: Implications for Computer System Design." *Journal of Systems and Software* 17, no. 1 (January 1992): 7–14.

Fujimoto, James G., Costas Pitris, Stephen A. Boppart, and Mark E Brezinski. "Optical Coherence Tomography: An Emerging Technology for Biomedical Imaging and Optical Biopsy." *Neoplasia* 2, no. 1–2 (Jan. 2000): 9–25. https://doi.org/10.1038/sj.neo.7900071.

Gilligan, Carol. *In a Different Voice: Psychological Theory and Women's Development*. Cambridge, MA: Harvard University Press, 1982.

"Global Study: 82% of People Believe Robots Can Support Their Mental Health Better Than Humans." Oracle News Connect, Oct. 7, 2020. https://www.oracle.com/news/announcement/ai-at-work-100720.html.

Grace, Katja, John Salvatier, Allan Dafoe, Baobao Zhang, and Owain Evans. "When Will AI Exceed Human Performance? Evidence from AI Experts." arXiv, May 3, 2018. https://arxiv.org/pdf/1705.08807.pdf.

Guizzo, Erico. "Telenoid R1: Hiroshi Ishiguro's Newest and Strangest Android." *IEEE Spectrum*, Aug. 1, 2010. https://spectrum.ieee.org/automaton/robotics/humanoids/telenoid-r1-hiroshi-ishiguro-newest-and-strangest-android.

Hafner, Katie. "A Robot That Coos, Cries and Knows When It Needs a New Diaper." *New York Times,* Nov. 16, 2002. https://www.nytimes.com/2000/11/16/technology/a-robot-that-coos-cries-and-knows-when-it-needs-a-new-diaper.html.

Hall-Flavin, Daniel K. "The Quality of Mercy." In *Spirituality and Deep Connectedness: Views on Being Fully Human*, edited by Michael C. Brannigan, 49–66. Lanham, MD: Lexington Books, 2018.

Hawkins, Andrew. "The World's First Robot Car Death was the Result of Human Error—And It Can Happen Again." *The Verge,* Nov. 20, 2019. https://www.theverge.com/2019/11/20/20973971/uber-self-driving-car-crash-investigation-human-error-results.

Heifetz, Ronald A., and Donald L. Laurie. "The Work of Leadership." *Harvard Business Review* 5, no. 1 (January-February 1997): 124–34.

Hertz, Noreena. *The Lonely Century: How to Restore Human Connection in a World That's Pulling Apart*. New York: Currency, 2021.

Hochman, David. "18 Weeks." *AARP Bulletin* 61, no. 10 (December 2020): 8–21. "Four Months that Left 54,000 Dead from COVID in Long-Term Care, The Oral History of an American Tragedy." *AARP* (December 3, 2020), https://www.aarp.org/caregiving/health/info-2020/covid-19-nursing-homes-an-american-tragedy.html.

Humphreys, Paul. *Extending Ourselves: Computational Science, Empiricism, and Scientific Method*. New York: Oxford University Press, 2004.

Iacoboni, Marco. *Mirroring People: The Science of Empathy and How We Connect with Others*. New York: Picador, Farrar, Straus and Giroux, 2008.

"'I'm Cheering for You': Robot Welcome at Tokyo Quarantine Hotel." *The Straits Times*, May 1, 2020. https://www.straitstimes.com/asia/east-asia/im-cheering-for-you-robot-welcome-at-tokyo-quarantine.

Ishiguro, Kazuo. *Klara and the Sun.* New York: Alfred A. Knopf, 2021.

Jewett, Christina. "'Lost on the Front Line': Tracks Health Workers Who Died of COVID-19." Interview with Steve Innskeep. NPR Transcript, April 8, 2021. Audio, 06:00. https://www.npr.org/transcripts/985253407.

Jewett, Christina, Shefali Luthra, and Melissa Bailey. "Federal Records Show Thousands of Desperate Pleas from Health Care Workers Seeking Better COVID Protective Gear." ABC News, June 30, 2020. https://abcnews.go.com/Health/federal-records-show-thousands-of-desperate-pleas-health-care/story?id=71530087.

Kenaan, Hagi. *The Ethics of Visuality: Levinas and the Contemporary Gaze.* Translated by Batya Stein. London: I.B. Tauris & Co., Ltd. 2013.

Kimura, Takeshi. "Masahiro Mori's Buddhist Philosophy of Robot." *Paladyn, Journal of Behavioral Robotics* 9, no. 1 (May 5, 2018): 71–82. https://doi.org/10.1515/pjbr-2018-0004.

Kincaid, Ellie. "One Year into the Pandemic, More Than 3,000 Healthcare Workers have Died of COVID-19." *Medscape*, March 11, 2021. https://www.medscape.com/viewarticle/947304.

Kleinman, Arthur. *The Illness Narratives: Suffering, Healing, and the Human Condition.* New York: Basic Books, 1988.

Kranzberg, Melvin. "Technology and History: Kranzberg's Laws." *Technology and Culture* 27, no. 3 (July 1986): 544–60. https://doi.org/10.2307/3105385.

Kundera, Milan. *Slowness.* Translated by Linda Asher. New York: HarperCollins, 1995.

Kurzweil, Ray. *The Singularity Is Near: When Humans Transcend Biology.* New York: Penguin Books, 2006.

Lange, Ansgar, and Ben Maruthappu. "Could Autonomous Car Technology and AI Transform Home Care for the Elderly?" IBM Think Blog, May 23, 2019. https://www.ibm.com/blogs/think/2019/05/could-autonomous-car-technology-and-ai-transform-homecare-for-the-elderly.

Lanzoni, Susan. *Empathy: A History.* New Haven, CT: Yale University Press, 2018.

Latour, Bruno. *Petites leçons de sociologie des sciences.* Paris: La Découverte, 2006.

Lee, Min Ho, Ho Seok Ahn, and Bruce A. MacDonald. "A Case Study: Robot Manager for Multi-Robot Systems with Heterogeneous Component-Based Framework." Australian Robotics and Automation Association paper. https://www.araa.asn.au/acra/acra2015/papers/pap139.pdf.

Lee, Paul S. N., Louis Leung, Venhwei Lo, Chengyu Xiong, and Tingjun Wu. "Internet Communication Versus Face-to-Face Interaction in Quality of Life Social Indicators Research." *Social Indicators Research* 100, no. 3 (February 2011): 375–89. DOI 10.1007/s11205-010-9618-3.

Lelkes, Orsolya. "Happier and Less Isolated: Internet Use in Old Age." *Journal of Poverty and Social Justice* 21, no. 1 (February 2013): 33–46.

Levinas, Emmanuel. *Entre Nous: Thinking of the Other.* Translated by Michael B. Smith and Barbara Harshav. New York: Columbia University Press, 1998.

Levinas, Emmanuel. *Ethics and Infinity: Conversations with Philippe Nemo.* Translated by Richard A. Cohen. Pittsburgh, PA: Duquesne University Press, 1985.

Levinas, Emmanuel. "Meaning and Sense." In *Collected Philosophical Papers*. Translated by Alphonso Lingis. Pittsburgh, PA: Duquesne University Press, 1987, 75–108.

Levinas, Emmanuel. *Otherwise Than Being or Beyond Essence*. Translated by Alphonso Lingis. Pittsburgh, PA: Duquesne University Press, 1998.

Levy, David. *Love and Sex with Robots: The Evolution of Human-Robot Relations*. New York: HarperCollins, 2007.

Lin, Patrick, Keith Abney, and George A. Bekey. *Robot Ethics: The Ethical and Social Implications of Robotics*. Cambridge, MA: The MIT Press, 2012.

Locsin, Rozzano C., and Hirokazu Ito. "Can Humanoid Nurse Robots Replace Human Nurses?" *Journal of Nursing* 5, no. 1 (2018). http://www.hoajonline.com/nursing/2056-9157/5/1.

Loeffler, John. "Should We Fear Artificial Intelligence?" *Interesting Engineering*, Feb. 23, 2019. https://interestingengineering.com/should-we-fear-artificial-superintelligence.

"Lost on the Frontline." *The Guardian*, April 8, 2021. https://www.theguardian.com/us-news/ng-interactive/2020/aug/11/lost-on-the-frontline-covid-19-coronavirus-us-healthcare-workers-deaths-database.

Lown, Bernard. *The Lost Art of Healing*. New York: Ballantine Books, 1996.

MacArthur Foundation. "Human Diagnosis Project." Accessed March 2021. https://www.macfound.org/press/semifinalist-profile/human-diagnosis-project.

MacDorman, Karl F., and Hiroshi Ishiguro. "The Uncanny Advantage of Using Androids in Cognitive and Social Science Research." *Interaction Studies* 7, no. 3 (2006): 297–337. http://www.macdorman.com/kfm/writings/pubs/MacDorman2006AndroidScience.pdf.

Malka, Salomon. *Emmanuel Levinas: His Life and Legacy*. Translated by Michael Kigel and Sonja M. Embree. Pittsburgh, PA: Duquesne University Press, 2006.

Master, Farah. "Meet Grace, the Healthcare Robot COVID-19 Created." *Reuters*, June 9, 2021, https://www.reuters.com/business/healthcare-pharmaceuticals/meet-grace-healthcare-robot-covid-19-created-2021-06-09/.

Mayor, Adrienne. *Gods and Robots: Myths, Machines, and Ancient Dreams of Technology*. Princeton, NJ: Princeton University Press, 2018.

Mazzotti, Massimo. "Algorithmic Life." *Los Angeles Review of Books*, Jan. 22, 2017. https://lareviewofbooks.org/article/algorithmic-life/.

McCann, Colum. *Letters to a Young Writer*. New York: Random House, 2017.

McDermott, Drew. "Why Ethics Is a High Hurdle for AI." Paper presented at 2008 North American Conference on Computing and Philosophy. Bloomington, IN, July 12, 2008.

"Mental Health and Psychosocial Considerations during the COVID-19 Outbreak." World Health Organization, March 18, 2020. Accessed April 2, 2020. https://www.who.int/docs/default-source/coronaviruse/mental-health-considerations.pdf?sfvrsn=6d3578af_2.

Merleau-Ponty, Maurice. "The Child's Relations with Others." In *The Primacy of Perception and Other Essays on Phenomenological Psychology, the Philosophy of*

Art, History and Politics. Translated by William Cobb, edited by James M. Edie (Evanston, IL: Northwestern University Press, 1964), 96–155.

Merleau-Ponty, Maurice. *Phenomenology of Perception*. Translated by Colin Smith. London: Routledge & Kegan Paul, 1962.

Mok, Kimberley. "Robot Passes a Medical Licensing Exam for the First Time Ever." *The Newstack*, Dec. 7, 2017. https://thenewstack.io/robot-passes-medical-licensing-exam-first-time-ever/.

Mountain Marketing, Inc. "Family and Health Care Near Term Markets." Mar. 11, 2013. Accessed Feb. 2021. https://www.geckosystems.com/investors/GeckoSystems-Family_and_Health_Care_Markets.pdf.

Muller, Jerry Z. *The Tyranny of Metrics*. Princeton, NJ: Princeton University Press, 2018.

National Society of Professional Engineers®. "Code of Ethics for Engineers." Accessed Nov. 28, 2020. http://www.mtengineers.org/pd/NSPECodeofEthics.pdf.

Nichols, Tom. *The Death of Expertise: The Campaign against Established Knowledge and Why It Matters*. New York: Oxford University Press, 2017.

Nietzsche, Friedrich. *Twilight of the Idols or, How to Philosophize with a Hammer*. Translated by Richard Polt. Indianapolis, IN: Hackett Publishing Company, Inc., 1997.

Noddings, Nel. *Caring: A Feminine Approach to Ethics and Moral Education*. Berkeley: University of California Press, 1984.

Nørskov, Marco, ed. *Social Robots: Boundaries, Potential, Challenges*. Surrey, UK: Ashgate Publishing Limited, 2016.

Nuland, Sherwin. *How We Die: Reflections of Life's Final Chapter*. New York: Alfred A. Knopf, 1994.

Nussbaum, Martha C. *Frontiers of Justice. Disability, Nationality, Species Membership*. Cambridge, MA; Belknap Press, Harvard University Press, 2006.

O'Connell, James J. *Stories from the Shadows*. Boston, MA: BHCHP Press, 2015.

O'Neill, Onora. *Autonomy and Trust in Bioethics*. Cambridge, UK: Cambridge University Press, 2002.

Ofri, Danielle. *Singular Intimacies: Becoming a Doctor at Bellevue*. New York: Penguin Books, 2003.

Osterholm, Michael T., and Mark Olshaker. *Deadliest Enemy: Our War against Killer Germs*. New York: Little, Brown Spark, 2017.

Panchal, Nirmita, Rabah Kamal, Cynthia Cox, and Rachel Garfield. "The Implications of COVID-19 for Mental Health and Substance Use." Kaiser Family Foundation, Feb. 10, 2021. Accessed April 2021. https://www.kff.org/coronavirus-covid-19/issue-brief/the-implications-of-covid-19-for-mental-health-and-substance-use/.

Peck, Mary Lou. "The Future of Nursing in a Technological Age: Computers, Robots, and TLC." *Journal of Holistic Nursing* 10, no. 2 (June 1, 1992): 183–91.

Pellegrino, Edmund D. "Apologia for a Medical Truant." In *The Philosophy of Medicine Reborn: A Pellegrino Reader*, edited by H. Tristam Englehardt, Jr. and Fabrice Jotterand, xiii–xvii. Notre Dame, IN: Notre Dame University Press, 2008.

Pellegrino, Edmund D. "Philosophy of Medicine: Should It Be Teleologically or Socially Constructed?" In *The Philosophy of Medicine Reborn: A Pellegrino*

Reader, edited by H. Tristam Englehardt, Jr. and Fabrice Jotterand, 49–61. Notre Dame, IN: Notre Dame University Press, 2008.

Pipher, Mary. *Another Country: Navigating the Emotional Terrain of Our Elders*. New York: Riverhead Books, 1999.

Plato. *Protagorus*. Translated by Benjamin Jowett and edited by Gregory Vlastos. Indianapolis, IN: The Bobbs-Merrill Company, Inc., 1956.

Postman, Neil. *Amusing Ourselves to Death: Public Discourse in the Age of Show Business*. New York: Viking Penguin Inc., 1985.

Prescott, Tony. "Me in the Machine." *New Scientist* 335, no. 3013 (March 2015): 36–39. https://doi.org/10.1016/S0262-4079(15)60554-1.

Rai, Sarakshi. "The Himalayas Are Visible from India for the First Time in 30 Years because of Covid-19 Lockdown." *Esquire, The Middle East*, April 12, 2020. https://www.esquireme.com/content/45334-the-himalayas-are-visible-from-india-for-the-first-time-in-30-years-because-of-covid-19-lockdown.

Reeves, Bryon, and Clifford Nass. *The Media Equation: How People Treat Computers, Television, and New Media Like Real People and Places*. Stanford, CA: Center for the Study of Language and Information, Stanford University, 2003.

Reiser, Stanley Joel. *Technological Medicine: The Changing World of Doctors and Patients*. New York: Cambridge University Press, 2009.

Ricoeur, Paul. *The Symbolism of Evil*. Translated by Emerson Buchanan. New York: Harper & Row, 1967

Ricoeur, Paul. *Time and Narrative*, Volume 3. Translated by Kathleen Blamey and David Pellauer. Chicago: University of Chicago Press, 1988.

Robertson, Jennifer. *Robo sapiens japanicus: Robotos, Gender, Family, and the Japanese Nation*. Oakland, CA: University of California Press, 2018.

"Robotic Cody learns to bathe." *Georgia Tech College of Engineering*, Nov. 11, 2010. https://coe.gatech.edu/news/2010/11/robotic-cody-learns-bathe.

Samuel, Sigal. "How to Help People during the Pandemic, One Google Spreadsheet at a Time." *Vox*, April 16, 2020. https://www.vox.com/future-perfect/2020/3/24/21188779/mutual-aid-coronavirus-covid-19-volunteering.

Sarles, Harvey. "The Genesis of Morality." *Religious Humanism* 41, no. 1 (September 2010): 43–55. http://huumanists.org/sites/huumanists.org/files/articles/Genesis%20of%20Morality%20-%20Sarles_0.pdf.

Sasangohar, F., B. Donmez, A.C. Easty, A. C, and P.L. Trbovich. "The Relationship between Interruption Content and Interrupted Task Severity in Intensive Care Nursing: An Observational Study." *International Journal of Nursing* Studies 52, no. 10 (October 2015) 1573–81.

Schüll, Natasha Dow. *Addiction by Design: Machine Gambling in Las Vegas*. Princeton, NJ: Princeton University Press, 2012.

Selzer, Richard. *The Whistler's Room: Stories and Essays*. Washington, DC: Shoemaker & Hoard, 2004.

Senju, Atsushi, and Mark H. Johnson. "Is Eye Contact the Key to the Social Brain?" *Behavioral and Brain Sciences* 33, no. 6 (2010): 458–59.

Shaw, Keith. "Tombot Robotic Service Dog Wins 2019 Pitchfire, Hearts of Audience." *Robotics Business Review*, Oct. 3, 2019. https://www.roboticsbusinessreview.com/events/tombot-robotic-service-dog-wins-2019-pitchfire-hearts-of-audience.

"Sir Luke Fildes the Doctor." Tate Gallery. Accessed March 2021. https://www.tate.org.uk/art/artworks/fildes-the-doctor-n01522.

Smiley, Lauren. "What Happens When We Let Tech Care for Our Aging Parents." *Wired*, Dec. 19, 2017. https://www.wired.com/story/digital-puppy-seniors-nursing-homes/.

Solvelight Robotics. "Genibo SD Companion Robot Dog." Accessed Jan. 2021. https://www.solvelight.com/product/dst-robot-genibo-robot-dog/.

Sone, Yuji. *Japanese Robot Culture: Performance, Imagination, and Modernity*. New York: Palgrave, 2017.

Sparrow, Robert, and Linda Sparrow. "In the Hands of Machines? The Future of Aged Care." *Minds and Machines* 16, no. 2 (2006): 141–61.

Sumagaysay, Levi. "Sony's Aibo Robotic Dog Can Sit, Fetch and Learn What Its Owner Likes." *The Mercury News*, Sept. 24, 2018. https://phys.org/news/2018-09-sony-aibo-robotic-dog-owner.html.

Tegmark, Max. *Life 3.0: Being Human in the Age of Artificial Intelligence*. New York: Vintage Books, 2017.

Thomas, Lewis. *The Youngest Science: Notes of a Medicine-Watcher*. New York: The Viking Press, 1983.

Thompson, Dana-Claudia, Madalina-Gabriela Barbu, Cristina Beiu, Lilliana Gabriela Popa, Mara Madalina Mihai, Mihai Berteanu, and Marius Nicolae Popescu. "The Impact of COVID-19 Pandemic on Long-Term Care Facilities Worldwide: An Overview on International Issues." *BioMed Research International* 2020, Article ID 8870249 (November 11, 2020): 1–7. https://doi.org/10.1155/2020/8870249.

Toombs, S. Kay. "The Role of Empathy in Clinical Practice." In *Between Ourselves: Second-Person Issues in the Study of Consciousness*, edited by Evan Thompson, 247–58. Thorverton, U.K.: Imprint Academic, 2001.

Topol, Eric. *Deep Medicine: How Artificial Intelligence Can Make Healthcare Human Again*. New York: Basic Books, 2019.

Tronto, Joan. *Moral Boundaries: A Political Argument for an Ethic of Care*. New York: Routledge, 1993.

Turkle, Sherry. *Alone Together: Why We Expect More from Technology and Less from Each Other*. New York: Basic Books, 2011.

Turkle, Sherry. *Reclaiming Conversation: The Power of Talk in a Digital Age*. New York: Penguin Press, 2015.

Tversky, Amos, and Daniel Kahneman. "Judgement Under Uncertainty: Heuristics and Biases." *Science* 185, no. 4157 (1974): 1124–1231.

United Nations. "COVID-19 Infections Rise, Delta Variant Spreads to 132 Countries." *UN News*, July 28, 2021. https://news.un.org/en/story/2021/07/1096572.

"U.S. Health Care from a Global Perspective, 2019: Higher Spending, Worse Outcomes?" *Commonwealth Fund Issue Brief*, Jan. 30, 2020. https://www.commonwealthfund.org/publications/issue-briefs/2020/jan/us-health-care-global-perspective-2019.

Vallor, Shannon. "Carebots and Caregivers: Sustaining the Ethical Ideal of Care in the 21st Century." *Journal of Philosophy and Technology* 24 (2011): 251–268.

Vallor, Shannon. *Technology and the Virtues: A Philosophical Guide to a Future Worth Wanting.* New York: Oxford University Press, 2016.

Van Beusekom, Mary. "COVID-19 Spread Freely Aboard USS Theodore Roosevelt, Report Shows." *CIDRAP News*, University of Minnesota, Center for Infectious Disease Research and Policy, October 1, 2020, https://www.cidrap.umn.edu/news-perspective/2020/10/covid-19-spread-freely-aboard-uss-theodore-roosevelt-report-shows.

van Wynsberghe, Aimee. "Designing Robots for Care: Care Centered Value-Sensitive Design." *Science and Engineering Ethics* 19, no. 2 (June 2013): 407–33. DOI: 10.1007/s11948-011-9343-6.

Verghese, Abraham. "Culture Shock—Patient as Icon, Icon as Patient." *New England Journal of Medicine* 359, no. 26 (Dec. 25, 2008): 2748–51.

Verghese, Abraham. "The Importance of Being." *Health Affairs* 35, no. 10 (October 2016): 1924–27.

Wachter, Robert. *The Digital Doctor: Hope, Hype, and Harm at the Dawn of Medicine's Computer Age.* New York: McGraw-Hill Education, 2015.

Wallach, Wendell, and Colin Allen. *Moral Machines: Teaching Robots Right from Wrong.* New York: Oxford University Press, 2009.

Walton, Kendall L. *In Other Shoes: Music, Metaphor, Empathy, Existence.* Oxford: Oxford University Press, 2015.

Wax, Jack. "Choreographed Lives: Twins Marie Robertson and Maggie Dethrow Share Their Love of Dancing." *Inside Columbia*, May 27, 2020, https://insidecolumbia.net/2019/11/21/choreographed-lives.

Westbrook, J. I., A. Woods, M.I. Rob, M., W.T. Dunsmuir, and R. O. Day. "Association of Interruptions with an Increased Risk and Severity of Medication Administration Errors." *Archives of Internal Medicine* 170, no. 8 (April 26, 2010): 683–90.

Whitby, Blay. "Do You Want a Robot Lover? The Ethics of Caring Technologies." In *Robot Ethics: The Ethical and Social Implications of Robotics*, edited by Patrick Lin, Keith Abney, and George A. Bekey, 233–48. Cambridge, MA: The MIT Press, 2012.

Wittgenstein, Ludwig. *Zettel.* Translated by G.E.M. Anscombe. Berkeley: University of California Press, 1970.

World Health Organization. "World Health Organization Coronavirus (COVID-19) Dashboard." Accessed July 28, 2021. https://covid19.who.int/.

Wysa. Accessed March 2021. https://www.wysa.io/.

Zaki, Jamil. "Catastrophe Compassion: Understanding and Extending Prosociality Under Crisis." *Trends in Cognitive Sciences* 24, no. 8 (August 2020): 587–89.

Zhang, Sheng, Meng Yuan Diao, Wenbo Yu, Lei Pei, Zhaofen Lin, and Dechang Chen. "Estimation of the Reproductive Number of Novel Coronavirus (COVID-19) and the Probable Outbreak Size on the Diamond Princess Cruise Ship: A Data-Driven Analysis." *International Journal of Infectious Diseases* 93 (April 2020): 201–4.

Index

ageism. *See* elders
agency, moral, 62, 76–77, 80, 100–101
aging. *See* death; the elderly
AIBO robotic dog (Sony, Japan), 27
air pollution, 97
algorithms:
    and caregiving, 39–41, 90, 103
    data-dependence, 33, 39, 57, 83
    defined, 39
    limits of, xxiii, xxv
    linguistic, 28
    See also artificial intelligence (AI); carebots
AliveCor (Mountain View, CA), Kardia electrocardiogram, 36–37
Allegory of the Cave (Plato), 46
Allen, Colin, 62
Alone Together (Turkle), 46
Amazon Alexa, 78
American Nurses Association, 63
Anders, Günther, 79
Angelucci, Adriano, 82
anthropocentrism, narcissism:
    and androids, 75–78
    and Western views of technology, 15–17
APACHE (Acute Physiology and Chronic Health Evaluation), 56–57

Apple Watch atrial fibrillation detector, 37
Aronson, Louise, 104–5
artificial intelligence (AI):
    and artificial general intelligence (AGI), 75
    and "as if" characteristics, 59–60
    and designed caring, 64
    expanding use of, xvi, 33
    and focus on the present, 12
    and incomplete replication of humanness, 12, 40–41
    integration with robotics, xvii
    medical applications, 33–37
    and robotic surgery, 34–35
    role of algorithms in, 39
    role in medical diagnosis, xxiv
    screen design and mode error, 48
    and self-consciousness, 64–65
    and simulations, 59
    and social interactions/empathy, 14–15
    superintelligence, self-programming, 59, 64
    voice platforms, 35
    See also medical diagnosis; medical technology
"as if" paradigm (Turkle), 59, 61, 70, 70–71n43, 88, 93

Asimov, Isaac, 65–66
Astro Boy, 4
Auris Health endoscopic robot, 35
automation bias/complacency, 50–51
Ayrton, Michael, 57–58, 106–7

Barcaro, Rosangela, 64
Baudrillard, Jean, 46
Bauerlein, Mark, 99
Bautista, Nestor, 7
Beck, Douglas, 35–36
Becker, Ernest, 57
Berger, Mayer, 10
Berkowitz, Avraham, 10
"in-betweenness" (*aidagara*), and true caring, 62–63
bioethics of caring, xix, 107–9
Birchenbough, Barbara, 7
"Blade Runner" (film, Scott), 4, 12
"Blade Runner 2049" (film, Villeneuve), 12
body language. *See* eye contact; face-to-face communication; presence, embodied
Boston Health Care for the Homeless Program, 31
the brain, 15
Bramsløw, Lars, 35–36
Brave New World (Huxley), 99
Breazeal, Cynthia, 47, 60
Broadbent, Elizabeth, 79–81
Brooklyn, NY, COVID-related deaths in, 10
Brooks, Robert, 25
Brynjolfsson, Erik, 33
Buber, Martin, 92
Bukimi no Tani (Mori). *See* Uncanny Valley (*Bukimi no Tani*)
Buoy Health Inc. (Boston), Symptom Checker tool, 36

Čapek, Karel, 3
Cambridge Medical Robotics (U.K.), "Versius" surgical robot, 35
carebots:
and absence of empathy, 88, 108
accepting, and the "as if" paradigm, 59, 93
agelessness of, 103
benefits and limits of, xxiv–xxv, 5–6, 11–12, 64, 90–91, 115–16
care.coach, 37–38
as companions, xxv, 15, 25–27, 58
design and development of, xvi, 58, 93
diversity of, 24–25
humanized, xxv, 75, 78–80, 100–101
and human-to-robot relationships, xvii–xix, 46–47
inability to actively listen, 107
inability to genuinely care, xxv, 5–6, 41, 61–64, 75
maximal vs. optimal use, 51
and moral agency, 61–62, 76–77, 101
and reduced human-to-human contact, 54, 67–68, 93
"self-consciousness," challenges raised by, 65
subjective human responses to, 83–84
as therapists, 26–28
too perfect, discomfort of, 79
and touch, 112–13
as trustworthy/consistent, xvii–xix, xxiii, 5–6, 11, 22–24, 29–32, 80–82, 98, 109–10
value-sensitive design, 101
care.coach (Wang and Deng), 37–38
caregiving:
and active listening, 106–7
benefits and limits of robots for, xxiv–xxv, 22–23, 100
capabilities approach, 63
caregiver shortages, xxii–xxiii, 24–26, 37, 100–101
and catastrophic compassion, 115
complexity/interdependence of, xxiii, 62–63
as a covenant between caregiver and the cared-for, 54, 77–78, 89–92

and empathy/embodied presence, x, xxvi, 56, 84–86, 104–10
genuine, characteristics of, xix, xxv–xxvi, 5, 40–41, 53, 56–57, 62, 91–92, 101, 115–16
as moral responsibility, 64, 90, 101–2
and obsession with speed, 53
purpose of, 40–41
and recognizing the singularity of the other, 90–91, 101–3
taking care of vs. caring about, xxv, 41, 60, 62, 115
and taking the first step, 90
and tender loving care, 63–64
and touch, 89, 110–13
and Western denial of death, 58
See also carebots; face-to-face communication; listening; medical technology
Carr, Nicholas, 50–51, 78
Cassell, Eric, 47, 55
Center for Infectious Disease Research and Policy (CIDRAP) pharmacist study, xx
Cera Care/IBM Research U.K., LiDar monitoring technology, 24–25
Chalmers, David, 15–17, 83
Chang, Ted, 34
chatbots, 27–28
China, AI development in, 32–33
chronicity, 22–23, 104
The Circle (Eggers), 28
Clara Maass Medical Center, Belleville, NJ, 7
Clark, Andy, 15–17, 83
Cockburn, Steve, 9
Cody (robotic nurse), 24
cognition
human, replicating, 14–15
human vs. machine, 16–17
relationship with behavior, 83
relationship with feeling, 87
Cohen, John, xxiii
Cohen, Stanley, 78
communication:

as characteristic of genuine care, xxvi
computer-mediated vs. face-to-face, 85
and eye contact/body language, 74–75
and *le dire* (the saying), 111
and role of the face, 73–74
and rules of interaction, 74
verbal, enhancement through gesture, 84
See also facial communications
connectedness, connectivity vs., 54
consciousness, challenges of understanding, 65
contagion. *See* COVID-19 pandemic; nursing homes/long-term care facilities
The Courage to Fail (Fox and Swazey), 13
COVID-19 pandemic:
and acclimation to technology, 4–5
and dying alone, 10
early spread, xii
environmental impacts, 97–98
fatality rates, xiii, 32
frontline workers, 9
and future pandemics, xxiv
global death toll, 8–9
and the homeless, 31
ICUs and surge capacity, 31–32
impact on nursing homes, xv–xvi
and increased mental health issues, 21
interactions and relationships during, 3
need to sustain interconnection, 22
in prisons, 30
quarantine/confinement, 28
remote communications during, 17
reproductive numbers (ROs) associated with, 30
social collateral damage, 10
and supply shortages, xiii–xiv, 7
toll on healthcare workers, 6–7

critical thinking vs. societal relativism, 99
Crozier, Brett, 29
Csepregi, Gabor, 73–74

Daedalus myth, xxvi, 21, 51, 57–58, 97, 106, 113, 115
Dall'Agnol, Darlei, 54
Damiano, Luisa, 15–17, 108
Dasarobot/Dasatech, South Korea, Genibo robotic dog, 26
Dautenhahn, Kerstin, 26
da Vinci Surgical System, 34
death:
    and dying and grieving alone, 10–11
    of healthcare workers from COVID, 7–10
    predicting, value for families and caregivers, 39–40
    Western denial and fear of, 57–58, 105
    See also COVID-19 pandemic; the elderly
deep medicine, 34
DeepMind (Google), AlphaZero AI system, 59
deep neural networking (DNN), 33, 35–36, 39
DeJesus, Vincent, 7
Deng, Shuo, 37
The Denial of Death (Becker), 57
dependability:
    acting dependably vs. being dependable, 61
    as a choice, 6
    and showing vs. being, 109
Designing Sociable Robots? (Breazeal), 47
Deutsch, Helene, 59, 70–71n43
Diamond Princess cruise ship, 29–30
Dick, Philip K., 4, 12
The Digital Doctor (Wachter), 47–48
the disabled, special needs, 52–53
DNN. *See* deep neural networking (DNN)

Do Androids Dream of Electric Sheep? (Dick), 4, 12
"The Doctor" (painting, Fildes), 10
Dumouchel, Paul, 15–17, 108

Edelman, Toby, xv
Eggers, Dave, 28
Ehrlich, Paul, 47
elders:
    abuse of, 101
    ageism, xv–xvi, 21–22, 51, 103, 105
    and aging as a pathology, 52
    and the denial of death, 58
    and the experience of aging, 103–5
    isolation, need for human contact, 93
    in Japan, 22, 53–54
    percentages of by country, 22
    roles for carebots, 53–54, 63
electrocardiogram apps, 36–37
electronic health records (EHRs), 2, 40, 47
emotions:
    of carebots, 12
    conveying physically, 74–75
    emoji, 73–74
    and eye contact, 56
    and life experience, 103
    and the mind, 17
    and mirror neurons, 87–88
    relationship with cognition, 86
    simulated by robots, 60, 65, 98–99
empathy:
    carebot potential for, 108
    communicating face-to-face, 85–86
    as a concept, 86
    and deep empathy, 34
    and embodied presence, 105–6
    and experiencing otherness, 88
    and genuine caring, xxvi, 4
    link to imagination, xviii
    and mirror neurons, 86
    See also caregiving; eye contact; face-to-face communication
EMRs. *See* electronic health records (EHRs)

Epimetheus, 45, 97
ethics. *See* bioethics
Experiment Perilous (Fox), 12–13
extended mind theory, 15–17, 83
eye contact:
   defined, 69n35
   importance, 56, 74–75
   in Western societies, 80

the face:
   and assumptions about agency, 80
   familiar, appeal of, 93
   and perceptions of
     humanness, 82, 88–89
   seeing genuinely as key to
     caregiving, 80, 91–92
   and the smile, 82
   See also *le Visage*
face-to-face communication:
   basic expressions, 87
   and communicating caring, 56
   complexity of, 73
   and *emoji*s, 73
   and empathy, 86
   and face proximity/distancing, 79
   and facial paralysis/
     immobility, 86–87
   importance, 74–75
   and infant moral development, 74
   and moral responsibility for
     each other, 89
   and the power of gesture, 84
   simulation of by robots,
     75, 78, 80–81
   subtlety of, 87
   See also body language; empathy;
     eye contact; *le visage* (the face)
family caregivers. *See* caregiving
Fèvre, Eric, xx
In the Field (Fox), 13–14
Fildes, Luke, 10
Fischer, Jeremy, 77
forty (*quaranta*), symbolism of, 28
Fox, Renée C., 12–13
Fredericks, Rachel, 77

Friedman, Batya, 56
Fukushima Daiichi Nuclear Power
   Station meltdown and robots, 23

GeckoSystems, U.S., 24
Geminoid (Ishiguro), 75–77
Genibo robotic dog (Dasarobot, South
   Korea), 26
Georgia Institute of Technology, 24
Gesture:
   as communication, 105
   as embodiment of caring, 84–85
   and parental care, 74
   robot simulation of, 65, 80
Gilligan, Carol, 62
Gods and Robots (Mayor), 73
Goffman, Erving, 73–74
Grand Princess cruise ship, COVID-19
   outbreak, 29
Graziani, Pierluigi, 82
Greek art, facial depictions in, 73
grieving and dying alone, 10–11. *See*
   also death

Hall-Flavin, Daniel, 109
hands and feet:
   human, unique qualities, 77
   in humanlike robots, 75, 83–84
   See also touch
Hanson Robotics, Hong Kong, Sophia
   and Grace, 75
healthcare system:
   content vs. context, 52–53
   costs of, 8
   cracks exposed by COVID
     pandemic, 9
   in high-income countries, 8
   and inadequate clinical training, 104
   positive uses for robots, 2, 23, 33
   and uncertainty in diagnosis, 12–14
   US, comparison with other
     systems, 7–8
   Western obsession with speed, 53
   See also caregiving; medical
     diagnosis; medical technology;

nursing homes/long-term care facilities
healthcare workers:
   and caregiving tasks vs. empathic caring, 41
   and the complexity of nursing, 63
   shortages of, xx, 6, 9, 28, 37
   toll of COVID pandemic on, 6–10
   value of AI assistance, 32
   See also caregiving; nursing homes, long-term care facilities
Hegel, Georg Michael Friedrich, 2
Heidegger, Martin, xxi, 77
Heifetz, Ronald, 3
Hephaestus, 1, 45, 73, 97. *See also* Pandora; Talos
"Her" (film, Jonze), 46
Hesiod, 45–46
history, lessons from, xxi–xxii
homeless people, special needs, 31
hope in the Pandora story, 45–46
Human Diagnosis Project (Human Dx app), 36
humans:
   and agency, 61
   ambiguity, uncertainty of, 55
   and anthropocentrism, 1, 15–17, 59–60
   caring as attribute of, 62
   disease vulnerabilities, 40
   and embodiment, 74, 79–80
   essential singularity/uniqueness of, 75, 101–3, 106–7
   as fallible, xxii, 40
   and fear of death, 57–58
   and genuine caring, xxv–xxvi, 5
   and the me-focused mindset, 99
   moral agency, 76–77
   as "natural cyborgs," 15
   as natural toolmakers, 51
   need for recognition, 77–78
   programming to accept robotics, 1, 38–39, 58, 93
   subjective responses to the unfamiliar, 82–84
   uncritical trust in technology, xxii, 3, 28, 50–52, 55–58, 77, 80–82, 98–99, 104
   and Zeus's gift of justice, 45
   See also caregiving; human-to-human relationships; human-to-robot relationships; presence, embodied
human-to-human relationships:
   and "in-betweenness" (*aidagara*), 62–63
   and caring, xxv, 62
   during COVID-19 pandemic, 3
   and embodied presence, 10–11
   and empathy, 85–86
   and full connectedness, 54
   and gesture, 79, 84–85
   imago Dei, 77–78
   importance, 21–22, 54, 63
   and interconnectedness/interdependence, 17, 62–63
   nuance and complexity in, xxiii
   and online learning, 69n22
   proximity/distancing, 79
   and robots as companions, xxv, 15, 25–27, 58
   and social isolation, xviii, 22
   and subjective responses to the unfamiliar, 83–84
   and touch, 110–11
   and transcendent encounter with the other, 89, 111
   See also caregiving; face-to-face communication; presence, embodied
human-to-robot relationships:
   "active externalism," 83
   and anthropomorphizing, 59–60
   automation bias/complacency, 50–51
   and the butterfly effect, 115
   coevolution of, 108
   and cognition, 14–17
   and desire for magic bullets, 47
   dichotomizing, as false, 93
   as dynamic, 83

and emphasis on speed, 53
and the "extended mind," 15–17, 83
and finding balance/poise, 37, 98–100
and human duty to not harm, 100
and humanized components, 75–76, 80
and human needs, desires, values, 4, 99–100
impacts on human-to-human relationships, xix, xxv–xxvi, 113–14
lessons from the past, xxi–xxii
and machine companionship, xxv, 15, 25–27, 58
and mechanistic uncaring activities, 77
as a merging/melding, 92
and moral agency, 76–77, 100–101
overdependence on machines, 33, 51, 58
and preference for robots, 46–47
revisiting assumptions about, 17, 77–79
subjectivity of human responses, 83–84
and the Uncanny Valley metaphor, 76–83
See also carebots
Humphreys, Paul, 15–16
the hyperreal, 46

Iacoboni, Marco, 86–88
IBM Watson supercomputer, xvi–xvii, 16, 25, 33
Icarus, 97, 113
iCub robots, 64–65
iFlyTek/Tsinghua University, Xiaoy robot, 32–33
illness-as-lived, xviii, 75
imagination, creativity:
  and the Daedalus legend, 21
  dulling of by technology, 99
  and empathy, xviii, xxiv
  and imagining the distant future, xxi

replicating robotically, xviii
immediacy, the quick fix, 52–53
intent and true care, 5–6
interconnection:
  and the cognitive domain, 16–17
  genuine, 3
  maintaining, 22
  See also caregiving; face-to-face relationships
Intuition:
  and caring, 63
  and empathy, xviii, 86
  and medical diagnosis, 104
iPatients, 40, 55
iRobi and Cafero robots (Yujin Robot), 24
iRobot, Cambridge, MA, 25
Ishiguro, Hiroshi, 24, 26, 75–77
Ishiguro, Kazuo, xvii–xviii 81

Japan:
  emoji and Japanese language conventions, 73–74
  principles for living with robots, 66–67
  quarantine robots, 98
  role of robots in culture of, 4, 25–26, 53
  "Silver Tsunami," 22
  sociable robots, 25
Jennie robotic therapy dog (Tombot, California), 26
Johnson, Mark, 56
Johnson & Johnson, Verb Surgical, 35
Jonze, Spike, 46

kami (spirit), 4
Kardia (AliveCor, Mountain View, CA), 36–37
KASPAR robotic therapy for children (Dautenhahn, U.K.), 26
Khan, Peter, 56
Kimura, Takeshi, 92–93
Kirzweil, Ray, 101–2
Kismet robot (MIT Labs, Breazeal), 60

Klara and the Sun (Ishiguro), xvii–xviii, 26, 81, 92
Kleinman, Arthur, 22–23, 41, 104
Kohlberg, Lawrence, 62
Kranzberg, Melvin, 99–100
Kundera, Milan, 53

Laennec, René, 113
Lange, Ansgar, 25
Latour, Bruno, 15
le dire (the saying; Levinas), 111
Lefkovsky, Eric, 39
Levinas, Emmanuel, xxi, xxv, 88–90, 111
le visage (the face; Levinas):
 embodied, and the irreducibility of the Other, 81
 engaging with, 90
 meaning of for human caring, xxv
 as revealer of vulnerability, 89
Levy, David, 58, 92
LiDar technology, 24–25
Life 3.0 (*Tegmark*), 51
Life Care Center, Kirkland, WA, xiii
Lifton, Robert Jay, xxvi
Lipps, Theodore, 86
listening, active, xviii, xxvi, 27, 106–8, 116
Liu Qingfeng, 32
Loeffler, John, 64
Lolley, Allison, xiii
Lorenz, Edward Norton, 115
"Lost on the Frontline" (*The Guardian* and Kaiser Health News), 9
Love and Sex with Robots (Levy), 58, 92
Lucid Robotic System (Neural Analytics, Inc. Los Angeles), 35

"magic bullet," 47
manga (comics), Astro Boy, 4
Maruthappu, Ben, 25
Matsushita, Japan, Wandakun robot, 26–27
Mayer, Stephan A., 35
Mayor, Adrienne, 73

The Maze Maker (Ayrton), 57–58, 106
Mazzotti, Massimo, 38–39
McAfee, Andrew, 33
McCann, Colum, 88
McCarthy, John, 33
McDermott, Drew, 61
Medea, 1
media equation, 78, 100
Media Lab, MIT Jibo robot, 47
medical diagnosis:
 and active listening, 107
 AI-assisted, 35
 and cognitive bias, 40
 complexity and uncertainty of, 12–14
 decision support tools, 56–57
 and deep neural networking; 33, 35–36, 39
 and human fallibility, 40
 IBM Watson supercomputer, xvi–xvii, 16, 25, 33
 and intuition, 104
Medical Humanities and Bioethics curriculum, University of Missouri, x, 108–9
medical technology:
 and adverse outcomes, 48–50
 alarm fatigue, 49
 and artificial voice platforms, 36
 "black-boxed," 39
 consumer technologies, 36–37
 and deep neural networking, 39
 and doctor-patient relationships, 55, 111–13
 electronic health records (EHRs), 2, 40, 47
 growing role in health care, 2–3, 55
 interactive, 36, 73
 and iPatients, 40, 55
 maximal vs. optimal use, 51
 and medical errors, 47–50
 and medications, 104
 pharmacy-technician robot, 50
 and pragmatism, 35–36, 51, 63, 101
 robotic surgery, 34–35
 and self-diagnosis tools, 36

stethoscope, 113
uncritical dependence on, xxii, 3, 28, 50–52, 55–58, 77, 80–82, 98–99, 104
and unnecessary diagnostic procedures, 55–56
See also carebots; caregiving
The Merchant of Venice, 109
Merleau-Ponty, Maurice, xxv, 79, 89
mind and the cognitive domain, 15–17
Mirroring People (Iacoboni), 86
mirror neurons, 86
Mitsubishi, South Korea, Wakamaru carebot, 24
Mobile Service Robots (MSRs; GeckiSystems), 24
mode errors, 49
Modfly, Thomas, 29
Monroe, LA nursing home conditions, xiii
Moor, James, 61
Moral Boundaries (Tronto), 101
morality:
 and agency, 62, 76–77
 and caring, 64, 90, 100–101
Mori, Masahiro, 76–77, 84, 92
My Real Baby animatronic doll (iRobot, Cambridge, MA), 25
myth:
 as fundamental truth, 1
 and mythic time, 2
 and unheeded warnings, xxiv, 97
 and visions of human potential, xxiv

Nass, Clifford, 78 100
National Society of Professional Engineers (NSPE), Code of Ethics, 67
naturalness, defining, 83
Neural Analytics Inc. (Los Angeles), 35
1984 (Orwell), 99
Niobid Painter, 73
Noddings, Nel, 5, 62
Norvig, Peter, 48
Nuland, Sherwin, 14

nursing homes/long-term care facilities:
 fatality rates, xiii
 lack of PPE or training, xiii–xiv, 7
 loneliness in, 60
 networks and interconnections among, xiv–xv
 spread of COVID-19 in, xiii–xvi
 understaffing, xv
 vulnerabilities of patients in, xiv
 See also healthcare workers
Nussbaum, Martha, 52–53, 63

objects, anthropomorphizing, 78, 100
Occupational Safety and Health Administration (OSHA), 7–8
O'Connell, Jim, 31
Ofri, Danielle, 102, 110
"old person" as a term, 103
Oldstone, Michael B., xx
O'Leary, John, 107
Olshaker, Mark, xx
O'Neill, Onora, 109–10
online learning, 69n22
Organization for Economic Co-operation and Development (OECD), 8
Osaka University, Japan, Ishiguro's robots, 24
Osterholm, Michael T., xx
the Other:
 and empathy, 85–86, 108
 encountering essence of, 92
 face of, as both concealing and revealing, 90
 recognizing singularity and transcendence of, 88–89
Otherwise than Being (Levinas), 89

pandemics, increasing incidence of, xx. *See also* COVID-19 pandemic
Pandora, 45–46, 73, 97, 114
"Parable" (Selzer), 91
Paracelsus, 104
"Paro" (baby harp seal) robot, xvii, 25
Parsons, Talcott, 12

Peck, Mary Lou, 63
Pellegrino, Edmund D., 107
Pepper (Tokyo hotel robot), 98
Perry, Sherry, xiv
Pesto, Marlyn, 109
Peter Bent Brigham Hospital, Boston, medical uncertainty study, 12–13
pharmacy-technician robot, 50
phenotyping, deep, 34
Pipher, Mary, 116
Plato, 45
poise, 100, 105–6
Postman, Neil, 98–99
pragmatism and using technology, 35–36, 51, 63, 100
pratityasamutpada. See interconnectedness
Prescott, Tony, 64–65
presence, embodied:
 and gesture, 84–85
 and genuine caring, x, xxvi, 3
 as key aspect of caregiving, 10–11
 as key to caregiving, 105–10
 and relationship, xxv
 replicating robotically, xviii
 and touch, 110
prisons, COVID infection rates, 30
Prometheus, xxiv 17, 45, 57, 97
Protagoras (Plato), 45

Quammen, David, xx
quarantine, as a term, 28–29

Reclaiming Conversation (Turkle), 59
Reeves, Byron, 78, 100
Reiser, Stanley Joel, 113
relationships. *See* carebots; human-robot relationships; human-to-human relationships
reliable, acting vs. being, 6, 61
reproductive number (R0), 30
Republic (Plato), Allegory of the Cave, 46
ReThink Robotics cobot, 75
retinal imaging, 33

RIBA II (Robot for Interactive Body Assistance), 53
Ricoeur, Paul, 1–2
the Riddle, 12–14, 40, 107
Robertson, Jennifer, 25, 76, 84, 92
Robo Sapiens Japanicus (Robertson), 25
Robots:
 and acting "as if" they have knowledge, 59
 androids, 75–78
 benefits of, 4, 23
 consistent performance of, xxiii
 dark side, 4–5
 diverse types of, 3–4
 ethically developed, value-sensitive, 67, 101
 "faces" on, and trustworthiness, 80–81
 harming, 66
 inability to laugh, blush, or commit suicide, xxiii
 Japanese laws for living with, 66–67
 for "love" and sex, 58
 moral status, 100–101
 origin of term, 3
 "self-conscious," 64–65
 and too-human robots, 81–82
 utility of, 47
 See also carebots; human-robot relationships; medical technology
Robots and Empire (Asimov), 66
Robotto no iru kurashi (Living with Robots), 66–67
Rochin, Rodrigo, 37–38
Rogers, Brandon, 7
Rossi, Maria Grazia, 82
rough sleepers, special needs, 31
"R.U.R." (Čapek), 3–4

Salvarsan ("magic bullet"), 47
Sarles, Harvey, 74
The Second Machine Age (Brynjolfsson and McAfee), 33
seeing/gaze behavior, 80

self-awareness, efforts to
  program, 64–65
self-diagnosis, AI tools for, 36–37
Selzer, Richard, 91
Sen, Amartya, 63
Senju, Atsushi, 56
Shaffer, David, 34
Shibata, Takanori, xvii, 25
singularity of human being, 101–3
Siri/Alexa, responses to questions, 59
Sirridge, Marjorie and William, 108–9
skin cancer detection, 33
Slack, Warner, xxii
Slowness (Kundera), 53
Smiley, Lauren, 37
smiling, physiology of, 82
SoftBank, Pepper robot, 98
SONY Japan, AIBO robotic dog, 27
Sparrow, Robert and Linda, 68
stroke diagnosis, AI-assisted, 35
Sunrise Hospital and Medical Center, Las Vegas, 7
Supersizing the Mind (Chalmers), 83
supply shortages, xiii–xiv, 7
surgery, robotic, 34–35
Suzuki, Hiroko, 91
Swazey, Judith, 13
Symptom Checker (Buoy Health, Boston), 36

Talos (first robot), 1–2
technology/machines:
  acclimation to during the COVID pandemic, 4
  anthropomorphizing of, 59
  balancing benefits and detriments, xxv–xxvi, 98, 113
  Cassell's definition, 47
  and false sense of autonomy, 58
  growing role of, 4, 33, 99
  lure of, 28, 52–53
  as non-neutral, 101
  as "quick fixes," xix, 53–54
  as tools, 15, 51, 58, 98, 100
  uncritical trust of, xxii, 3, 28, 50–52, 55–58, 77, 80–82, 98–99, 104
  See also artificial intelligence (AI); human-to-robot relationships; medical technology
Tegmark, Max:
  on artificial general intelligence (AGI), 75
  on attributing humanness to robots, 80
  on concerns about mortality, 58
  and freedom from biological determinism, 51
  on self-improving machines, 59
Telenoid R1 android (Osaka University, Japan), 24
Tempus Labs, use of DNNs, 39
Tetsuro, Watsuji, 62–63
therapy robots, 25–28
Thomas, Lewis, 112
Three Laws of Robotics (Asimov), 65–66
Tombot (Santa Clara, California), robotic therapy dog, 26
Toombs, Kay, xviii
Topol, Eric, xvi–xvii, 34, 40
Touch:
  as communication, 35, 111–13
  and healing, xvii, 63, 89, 91–92, 102, 104, 110, 112–13
  human vs. robot, 3, 17, 47, 74, 105
Tronto, Joan, 60, 101, 115
Trust:
  and the caregiver's touch, 110
  and faces on robots, 80–81
  of robots, as fundamental, 109
  uncritical, in technology, xxii, 3, 28, 50–52, 55–58, 77, 80–82, 98–99, 104
Turkle, Sherry:
  "ELIZA" effect, 60–61
  "as if" paradigm, 59, 70–71n43, 88
  on the "robotic moment," 46
Tversky, Amos, 40

Uncanny Valley (*Bukimi no Tani*), 76–83
Uncertainty:
   and the appeal of medical technologies, 57–58
   and cognitive biases, 40
   and deep neural networks, 39
   intolerance for, xxiii, 51–52, 54–55
   types of in medical decision-making, 12–14
usefulness, confusion with value, 51, 66
U.S.S. *Theodore Roosevelt*, COVID-19 outbreak aboard, 29

Vallor, Shannon, xvi, 46
value-sensitive design, 101
Van Wynsberghe, Aimee:
   on limits of robotic care, 65
   on touch and trust, 110
   value-sensitive design, 101
Verb Surgical robot (Google & Johnson & Johnson), 35
Verghese, Abraham, 55, 105–6
"Versius" surgical robot (Cambridge Medical Robotics, UK), 35
Villeneuve, Denis, 12
voices, computerized:
   acceptance of voices, 78
   therapy robots, 26–28
   for the visually impaired, 36

Wachter, Robert, 47–49
Wakamaru (Mitsubishi carebot), 24
Wallach, Wendell, 62
Walton, Kendall, 87
Wandajun (koala) robot (Matsushita, Japan), 26–27
Wang, Victor, 37
Weizenbaum, Joseph, 60
What Is Called Thinking" (Heidegger), 77
Whitby, Blay, 58
Wittgenstein, Ludwig, 84
Woebot Health, chatbot therapy, 27
World Health Organization, 21–22
Wuhan, China, hospital robots, 98
Wysa chatbot therapy, 27

Xenex Disinfection Services (U.S.) decontamination robots, 98
Xiaoy ("little doctor") medical robot, 32–33, 98

The Youngest Science (Thomas), 112
Yujin Robot, South Korea, 24

Zaki, Jamil, 115
Zeus, 1, 45, 73

About the Author

Throughout his career, Michael C. Brannigan (Ph.D., Philosophy, M.A., Religious Studies, University of Leuven, Belgium) has been actively engaged in healthcare ethics. The former Pfaff Endowed Chair in Ethics and Moral Values at The College of Saint Rose in Albany, New York continues to teach Intercultural Bioethics as Adjunct Professor at the Alden March Bioethics Institute, Albany Medical College, and as Adjunct Professor in the Department of Philosophy, Salve Regina University, Newport, Rhode Island. Born in Fukuoka, Japan, his specialties embrace Asian philosophies, ethics, intercultural and medical ethics, and phenomenology. His books include *Healthcare Ethics in a Diverse Society*; *Ethical Issues in Human Cloning*, ed.; *Cross-Cultural Biotechnology*, ed.; *Cultural Fault Lines in Healthcare*, and *Japan's March 2011 Disaster and Moral Grit*. He speaks internationally and serves on the editorial board of *Communication and Medicine*. He also writes a monthly column for the *Albany Times Union* newspaper; see http://www.timesunion.com/brannigan/. He and his wife Brooke live in Wakefield, Rhode Island. For fun, he plays piano, ocean kayaks, studies martial arts and matters Japanese and Irish. His website is: https://www.michaelcbrannigan.com.

www.ingramcontent.com/pod-product-compliance
Lightning Source LLC
Chambersburg PA
CBHW020124010526
44115CB00008B/958